DEDICATION

This book is dedicated to:
My husband and children, who give my life meaning;
My parents, who shaped who I am;
My patients, who remind me why this work matters.

CONTENTS

HEALTHY LIVER HACKS

Follow the "water first" rule for a healthier liver.

Walk 10–15 minutes after every meal to prevent sugar spikes.

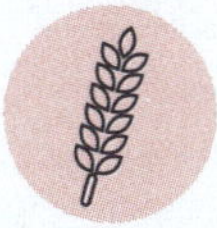

Consume whole grains to reduce fatty buildup in the liver.

Use cruciferous vegetables as natural detox partners.

175+ WAYS TO HEAL YOUR LIVER AND IMPROVE YOUR HEALTH!

SUPRIYA JOSHI, MD

ADAMS MEDIA
NEW YORK AMSTERDAM/ANTWERP LONDON TORONTO
SYDNEY/MELBOURNE NEW DELHI

Adams Media
An Imprint of Simon & Schuster, LLC
100 Technology Center Drive
Stoughton, MA 02072

First Adams Media trade paperback edition September 2026

Interior design by Sylvia McArdle
Images © Adobe Stock; 123RF

Manufactured in the United States of America

1 2026

Library of Congress Control Number: 2026939095.

ISBN 978-1-5072-2660-5
ISBN 978-1-5072-2661-2 (ebook)

INTRODUCTION

The liver is a multitasking powerhouse in your body, and its well-being is vital to your overall health—so it's time to protect it! The liver's main job is to filter your blood, removing toxins that are harmful to the body. But that's not its only role. It also stabilizes your blood sugar, stores essential nutrients, helps regulate hormones, and aids in breaking down the food you eat. If your liver is not functioning properly, it's impossible to live your best life. But with so much information out there, it can feel overwhelming to sort through it all and find the advice that's right for you. Enter *Healthy Liver Hacks*.

In this book, you'll find more than 175 hacks that will help streamline everything there is to know about protecting and improving your liver health. Because the liver can regenerate itself, it's possible for you to stop and reverse previous damage through these sustained healthy lifestyle changes. These hacks will help you understand and monitor your current liver function, choose the best dietary and lifestyle changes you can make to support your liver, and give you insight on how you can improve your liver health through prioritizing self-care and rest.

Whether you're hearing about the importance of liver health for the first time or you're looking for some actionable steps to help reverse liver damage, this book is here to keep your liver in the best possible shape!

HOW TO USE THIS BOOK

The hacks in this book have been designed to be simple to do and easy to incorporate into your daily life so you can prioritize your liver health every day. They have been divided into sections based on the facets of liver health they relate to, whether that be tests and metrics for assessing your liver health; ways to nourish your body and liver; physical actions you can start to strengthen your liver; in-depth knowledge on vitamins, supplements, and toxins that affect your liver; and ways to protect your liver through self-care and rest. You can read through these hacks sequentially or jump to the sections that feel most appropriate for you and your health goals.

But before you dive into implementing the hacks in this book, it's important to have a basic understanding of what the liver is. In Chapter 1, you'll get a wealth of knowledge about the role of the liver in your body, how it works, its many functions, and the diseases and conditions that can damage it. With this knowledge in hand, you'll be ready to explore the many ways you can monitor and boost your liver health to keep your body running in optimal shape.

HABIT STACKING

The goal of this book is not to overwhelm you but rather to make you aware of the many small opportunities for change that can help your liver health. One way you can jump-start that process is by utilizing "habit stacking." Habit stacking refers to adding some of this book's small healthy hacks onto each other according to your preferences, accessibility, and ability. When time is tight, remember the quick hacks in this book, and on those occasions when you have more time, you can add multiple hacks on top of each other to give yourself even more health improvements.

BONUS BENEFITS

When you implement the hacks in this book, you may also see improvements in other areas of your well-being, including your heart health, metabolic health, gut health, and energy levels. To help you understand which of these hacks can help which body systems, you'll find icons that call out the additional health benefits of each hack. These bonus benefits are:

Empowered Health: Progress happens when you know your baseline and you can compare your metrics. These hacks will help you understand your body's functions regarding your liver health and how to monitor them. That way you can better assess changes after taking the necessary interventions.

Gut Health: It should not be a surprise that the steps you take to improve your liver health will also improve your gut health. This means less bloating, better digestion, and overall health improvement.

Heart Health: These hacks provide a side benefit bonus of improving your cardiovascular fitness or heart health, which may also translate into improved lifespan.

Metabolic Health: Consistently implementing these habits will improve your blood sugar, insulin sensitivity, and weight.

Wellness and Energy: There is more to your wellness than your food and drink intake, and these hacks will help you consider how mindfulness, balance, exercise, rest, and good quality sleep all contribute to a healthier liver and lifestyle.

Chapter 1

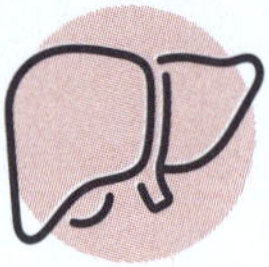

YOUR LIVER: YOUR BODY'S SILENT POWERHOUSE

Your liver is an amazing organ. It's your body's ultimate multitasker, a blend of a chemistry lab, storage warehouse, and power plant. It purifies your blood, processes your food, manages your hormones, and creates energy for you to live. It is also the only internal organ with the amazing power to regenerate itself. Interestingly, because you don't really "feel" your liver, like you can your pulse or heart rate, most people rarely think about it, and often abuse it without realizing. This chapter will help you understand your liver and its many vital functions. It will also explain the various diseases that can affect your liver so you can take the necessary steps to protect it.

THE STRUCTURE OF THE LIVER

Your liver is roughly the size of a football and is kept in place right under the diaphragm, which is the muscle that separates your chest and thorax from your abdomen. The liver sits under your right rib cage and beneath your right lung. A healthy liver is a deep reddish-brown color, which reflects its rich blood supply. The liver has two main blood vessels that feed it:

- The *hepatic artery* that brings oxygenated blood from the heart.
- The *portal vein* that carries nutrient-rich blood from your gut.

The liver is a very organized structure and is made up of four lobes; the right lobe is the largest, followed by the left lobe, then on the backside are the smaller caudate and quadrate lobes. These lobes contain millions of tiny hexagonal units called lobules, and each lobule holds strands of hepatocytes, which are the main working cells within the liver and are arranged much like spokes on a wheel. These cells are arranged around tiny central veins and channels that drain bile and process blood. Through this microscopic architecture, your liver filters, converts, stores, and synthesizes materials continuously.

FUNCTIONS OF THE LIVER

Your liver has many core functions, including producing bile, removing toxins from the blood, stabilizing blood sugar, and more. Let's explore each of these functions:

Produces Bile

Bile is your natural fat-digesting fluid; it breaks down fat in the body much like how dish soap breaks down grease on pans. Your liver cells make bile and then it travels down the tiny channels in your liver lobules to drain into the gallbladder. The gallbladder is a small pear-shaped organ beneath the liver where bile is stored and secreted

Anterior (front view)

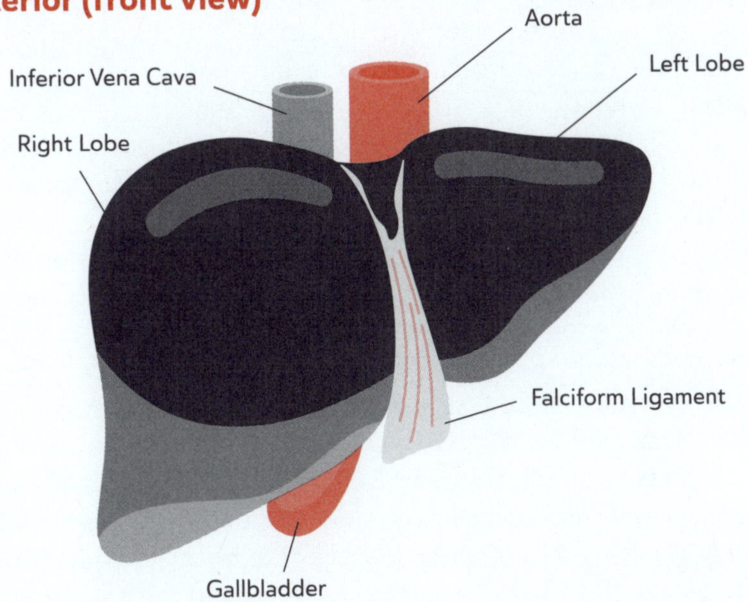

Posterior (back view)

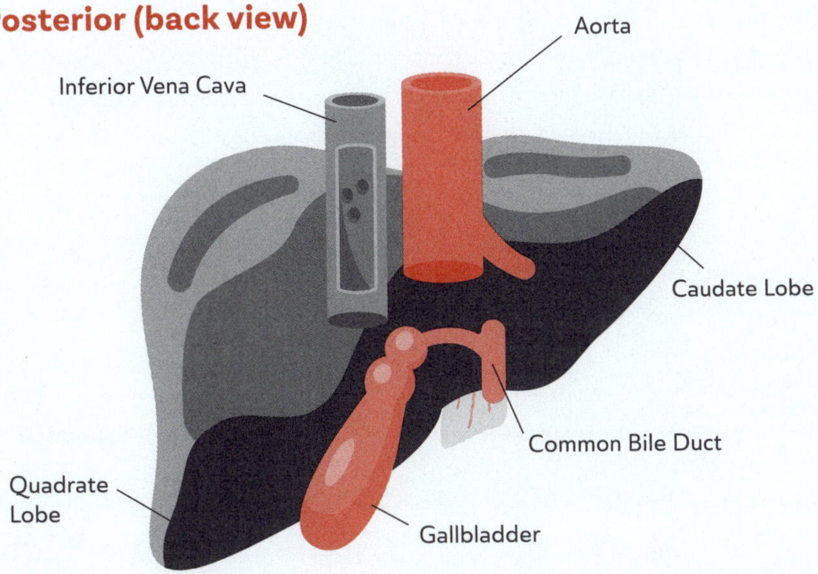

to help with digestion. It is also where tiny stones can form and, in some situations, cause pain in the right side of the body. When this happens, your gallbladder can become inflamed, and surgery may be needed to remove it to alleviate your discomfort and address or prevent infection. Even if your gallbladder is removed, bile can still travel down the common bile duct where it empties into your small intestine; it will just not be stored anywhere.

When you eat a fatty meal, bile is released, and this acts as a detergent to break down and digest the fat into elements your body can use. Bile is greenish-yellow and is made of bile acids, cholesterol, and pigments. Bile emulsifies fats, which is necessary for you to absorb vitamins A, D, E, and K. If you don't produce bile or your bile duct is blocked, your stool looks pale instead of brown, and your body isn't able to handle fats, which can lead to cramps, diarrhea, and malabsorption. Over time, this can also lead to malnutrition. The bile duct can be blocked by a passing stone that became impacted, bile duct inflammation, a scarred narrowing, or a tumor.

Removes Toxins from Blood

One of the primary functions of your liver is to detoxify your blood. Every drug, glass of wine, or processed snack you ingest enters your bloodstream and passes through your liver. Your hepatocytes then transform the harmful compounds into substances that can be carried away via the bile the liver produces. Bile enters the digestive tract, and the materials in it are eliminated through the digestive tract as feces.

Your liver's main purification system is the cytochrome P450 enzyme system, which deactivates toxins, medications, and hormones. This enzyme system exists in other tissues of the body as well, but the liver cells are the major site of P450 activity. While doing their job, sometimes these enzymes can produce toxic intermediates that can cause harm. When this system is further overwhelmed by alcohol, pollutants, or toxins, the liver suffers quietly until it can't keep up.

Stabilizes Blood Sugar

Your liver keeps your blood sugar steady. When you eat, any remaining glucose (sugar) your body doesn't need for fuel at that time is stored by the liver as glycogen (stored sugar molecules). In times of fasting, your liver breaks down the glycogen to release glucose and give you energy. Your liver can also convert protein and fats into energy when blood sugar levels run low. By doing this, the liver has a critical role in balancing blood sugar to prevent dangerously low levels (hypoglycemia) and dangerous sugar spikes (hyperglycemia). Having repeatedly high blood sugars leads to inflammation and injury of the tiny blood vessels throughout the body and subsequent damage of multiple organs.

Makes Important Blood Proteins

Your liver isn't just filtering; it's also building blood proteins. Blood proteins, also known as plasma proteins, are essential parts of your blood plasma and are fundamental to many of your body's processes, including transporting substances throughout the body, fighting infections, and ensuring blood clotting. Liver cells manufacture albumin, the most abundant protein circulating through your blood vessels. Albumin's main function is to prevent water in the bloodstream from leaking into surrounding tissues and causing swelling (also known as edema). In addition, liver cells synthesize almost all the proteins necessary for blood clotting factors, which are important so that you don't keep continuously bleeding from a simple cut. The liver also manufactures carrier proteins, which are necessary to transport hormones, metals, and drugs safely throughout the body. Without your liver being able to produce these essential proteins, you would experience swelling of the ankles and abdominal cavity, bruising of the skin, and the risk of uncontrolled bleeding.

Stores Essential Vitamins

Your liver is a nutritional vault. It holds vitamin A for vision, vitamin D for bones, vitamin B_{12} for nerves, and iron and copper for blood cell production. When your liver gets sick, these nutritional stores can be affected, and low levels may be detected. For example, chronic liver conditions can lead to iron-deficiency anemia, which can cause tiredness, weakness, and shortness of breath. Lab tests can specifically identify which vitamin or mineral deficiency has developed. By knowing this, the issue can be corrected and the symptoms improved.

Metabolizes Certain Hormones

When most people think of hormones, they often think of the thyroid and pancreas, but your liver is a central part of keeping hormonal health balanced. The liver is involved in the processing or breaking down of hormones such as estrogen, cortisol, thyroid hormones, and insulin. If the liver is not functioning optimally, hormone levels may fluctuate, possibly contributing to mood swings, irregular periods, fertility issues, weight gain, and even breast tenderness in both men and women.

Handles Cholesterol Production

Your liver produces 80 percent of your cholesterol, and it is important to acknowledge that cholesterol isn't a villain. Your body needs cholesterol to build cell membranes, make hormones like estrogen and testosterone, and produce vitamin D. A healthy liver keeps production balanced, but when it becomes overloaded with excess sugar, processed foods, or fat accumulation, that balance breaks down and cholesterol levels can creep in the wrong direction. Your liver produces VLDL, HDL, Apolipoprotein B (ApoB), and lipoprotein A, also called Lp(a). Your liver is the control center for cholesterol traffic, and it packages and ships cholesterol through your bloodstream using carriers called lipoproteins. When this system goes wrong, it becomes one of the most powerful drivers of heart disease.

LIVER CONDITIONS AND DISEASES

By now it should be clear to you that the liver does *a lot* for your health. It is also a very resilient organ and will keep working hard even when a large part of it is sick or damaged. Because of this resilience, it is often not apparent that the liver is struggling, and sometimes it is only discovered in advanced stages of liver disease or injury. Most liver diseases do not have any associated symptoms; however, in the "acute" phase of a sudden or extreme liver injury, there may be some typical symptoms that can occur in the case of viral infections, autoimmune liver disease, heavy alcohol intake, or drug injuries. These symptoms can include:

- Right-sided ache
- Nausea
- Reduced appetite
- Generalized itch
- Yellowing of the whites of the eyes (icterus)
- Yellowing of the skin (jaundice)
- Fatigue
- Fever
- Dark urine

While most liver diseases are silent, being aware they can exist is the first step to evaluating your situation and, in particular, your liver health. The hacks in this book can help address the issues caused by many of these diseases and, in some cases, help your liver heal from them. Let's take a look at some of the most common liver conditions afflicting people.

Fatty Liver Disease

The most common condition affecting the liver today is fatty liver disease. This condition was recognized in the 1980s and has since grown into a global epidemic. This condition was recently renamed metabolic dysfunction–associated steatotic liver disease (MASLD) to better characterize the underlying cause and be less stigmatizing. When more than 5 percent of your liver cells contain fat, the diagnosis of fatty liver is made. There are often no symptoms to suggest this disease is developing, but some people may experience an ache in their right side, feel sluggish, and experience weight gain. This condition develops when a diet is comprised of a high intake of sugar, refined carbohydrates, and processed food, and the consumed energy is subsequently turned into fat and stored inside liver cells. Genetics may also play a role in leading to more rapid progressive liver injury in some individuals.

Over time this condition causes inflammation (steatohepatitis) and scarring (fibrosis), which can occur in up to 30 percent of people with MASLD. When liver inflammation and fibrosis develop, the condition is called metabolic dysfunction–associated steatohepatitis (MASH), which is essentially an aggressive and progressive form of MASLD. Of this group with MASH, 10–25 percent of them can progress to liver cirrhosis. The individuals who are at higher risk of developing advanced liver fibrosis and cirrhosis are those with type 2 diabetes, hypertension, high cholesterol, and obesity.

The good news is that in most cases, to a certain point, this condition is reversible. Studies have repeatedly demonstrated that if an individual can lose 5–10 percent of their body weight, the liver fat, inflammation, and scarring can reverse. To achieve weight loss, it is advised that affected people reduce their intake of sugar, processed foods, and alcohol and that they incorporate regular exercise into their lives. In conjunction with lifestyle change, there are now some medications that have been shown to help people with MASH with stage 2 or 3 liver fibrosis.

Lifestyle changes are often easier said than done. Because these can be challenging to implement and many individuals simply may not know where to start, this book was designed to help with exactly that in mind: to teach the hacks in small, bite-sized morsels and help you achieve these goals.

Viral Hepatitis

While the liver is resilient, sometimes it can fall victim to viruses that can cause injury to it. There are five main viruses that can affect the liver, named hepatitis A, B, C, D, and E. These cause liver inflammation and in some rare cases can cause liver failure. Hepatitis B and C can also lead to chronic liver disease and even liver cirrhosis and liver cancer. Hepatitis A and E are acquired through contaminated food or water, whereas hepatitis B and C are primarily transmitted through contaminated blood and body fluids. Hepatitis D only occurs in people who are infected with hepatitis B. Some of these viral infections can be prevented by vaccination, and others have specific treatments and even cures.

Alcohol-Induced Liver Disease

Alcohol-induced liver disease remains the most common chronic liver disease worldwide. Alcohol is one of the most powerful toxins your liver has to handle. Each time you drink, your liver works to break down the alcohol. In the process, toxic by-products form that injure liver cells, trigger inflammation, and encourage toxic fat buildup. Over time, this repeated stress can lead to alcohol-induced liver disease. Though alcohol intake has been normalized in many parts of the world, we now know that any degree of alcohol intake is harmful to liver health. Chronic or regular alcohol intake can lead to liver cirrhosis and its complications, but it can also contribute to cardiovascular disease, pancreatitis, gastritis, mood disorders, addiction, poor sleep, dementia, and increased risk of multiple cancers.

Autoimmune Liver Disease

This is a category of conditions triggered when a person's own immune system accidentally injures their cells. More commonly known autoimmune conditions include autoimmune thyroid disease and type 1 diabetes. The liver can also be affected by antibodies produced by your body, and a family history of similar autoimmune conditions can increase your risk of being affected. Injury can occur directly to the hepatocytes, the microscopic bile ducts, or even the larger bile ducts running through the liver. While the symptoms of autoimmune liver disease vary from person to person, some people experience fatigue, belly discomfort, skin rash, joint pain, and yellowing of the skin and eyes. A diagnosis can be made by specific lab tests, imaging of the liver, and, in some cases, a liver biopsy. There is no cure for autoimmune disease, but there are treatments, including corticosteroids and immunosuppressants. If left untreated, a person could develop cirrhosis or even liver failure if the injury is severe.

THE STAGES OF CHRONIC LIVER DISEASE

If left untreated, all the liver conditions and diseases you just learned about will lead to chronic liver disease. Liver disease progresses through several stages before ending in liver failure. Those stages are:

1. Inflammation
2. Fibrosis
3. Cirrhosis
4. Liver failure

Let's take a look at each of those stages.

Liver Inflammation (Hepatitis)

When many people hear "hepatitis," they tend to think of the viral hepatitis mentioned earlier. However, the term "hepatitis" refers to any condition that causes inflammation in the liver, including the viral and nonviral conditions we previously discussed, like fatty liver disease, autoimmune disease, or alcohol-induced liver disease. Inflammation damages the liver; however, because of the liver's ability to regenerate itself, the damage from inflammation can be reversed. The problem is that when the liver inflammation becomes chronic, meaning the negative behaviors continue, the liver becomes overwhelmed and fibrosis develops.

Liver Fibrosis (Scarring)

Any condition that causes liver inflammation (such as viral infections, alcohol consumption, or fatty liver disease) can lead to liver scarring. Liver inflammation triggers a continuous repair cycle where damaged cells activate hepatic stellate cells (HSCs). These hepatic stellate cells typically store vitamin A and regulate liver homeostasis, but when they become activated by injured cells, they produce excessive collagen and form scar tissue (fibrosis). If inflammation persists, this scarring worsens, stiffening the liver, blocking blood flow, and eventually leading to cirrhosis, where the liver's architecture is permanently disrupted with regenerative nodules, severe fibrosis, and impaired function. Liver fibrosis stages describe the buildup of scar tissue in the liver, typically categorized from F0 (no fibrosis) to F4 (cirrhosis). Early stages (F1–F3) are often reversible with treatment of the underlying cause.

Reversal of liver fibrosis means reducing or eliminating the excess scar tissue in the liver, which happens by removing the underlying cause (like viruses, alcohol, or metabolic issues) and allowing liver cells to clear the scar, often involving the inactivation or elimination of HSCs that produce collagen. Traditionally, a liver biopsy was necessary to establish liver inflammation pattern and stage of fibrosis, but today, imaging and noninvasive testing can help your healthcare provider predict liver injury.

Cirrhosis

Cirrhosis is the scarring phase of the liver that results after years of injury. Previously soft, pink, healthy tissue turns hard and fibrotic, blocks blood flow through the tiny channels, and ultimately destroys the liver's ability to perform its necessary functions. Due to this high degree of liver cell destruction, a new liver may be the only hope for certain people. The majority of individuals with liver cirrhosis have no symptoms at all, although muscle wasting may be noted. Suggestions of cirrhosis may appear only on an abdominal ultrasound or CT scan, or certain lab tests may provide clues.

While the most common causes of liver cirrhosis worldwide are chronic alcohol intake and viral hepatitis, the truth is that any liver disease can lead to cirrhosis. While many patients with liver cirrhosis will not progress to liver failure, they are at risk of liver cancer, and the presence of cirrhosis may affect management of other medical problems outside of the liver. Once an individual has established cirrhosis, if the underlying causes of injury are not stopped, injury will progress, increasing the risk of liver failure and possible death.

Liver Failure

The term "liver failure" means your liver is shutting down and is unable to perform its basic jobs, such as filtering toxins, processing medicines and nutrients, making bile, and producing clotting proteins to keep you healthy. There are two different types of liver failure: acute and chronic.

- **Acute liver failure** happens fairly quickly, over weeks to days. It often happens when something overwhelms your liver, such as poison or a viral infection.
- **Chronic liver failure** (or acute-on-chronic) is when long-term liver disease worsens and becomes irreversible. The scar tissue is now preventing your liver from functioning.

The liver is famously known for its ability to regenerate itself. However, this regeneration ability holds only up to a certain point, and when it reaches its limits, the liver will deteriorate. Liver failure isn't rapid, but it is eventually fatal without a liver transplant. Signs and clues of liver failure are:

- Swelling of the ankles (edema)
- Distended abdomen (ascites)

- Yellowing of the eyes (icterus)
- Yellowing of the skin (jaundice)
- Dark urine
- Easy bruising
- Bleeding
- Muscle wasting
- Daytime sleepiness (encephalopathy)
- Nighttime wakefulness (encephalopathy)
- Confusion
- Musty, fruity breath (fetor)

Liver Transplant/Donation

If the person with liver failure is successfully placed on a transplant list, they are then ranked according to the severity of their illness and within their region of residence. Many can wait on the list for several months or even years for a liver from a traditional donor. The sad reality is that 9–20 percent of people on liver transplant waiting lists die because their disease has progressed too far and a new organ did not come in time. However, if they are fortunate, they have someone they know who is a blood-type match and willing to be a living donor.

A living donor is a person who donates part of their liver to help someone else who is in desperate need of a new liver. The most common type of "living" donor donation is when a healthy person donates the large right lobe of their liver, which equates to giving away 60–65 percent of their own liver (leaving the donor with 35–40 percent of their liver). Within 7 days the liver will begin to grow rapidly, both in the donor and the recipient. Within 6 to 8 weeks the liver regains 80 to 90 percent of its original volume, and by about 3 months, the liver's size and function are almost fully restored.

LOOKING FORWARD

Many people don't realize they may already be at risk for liver disease. Fortunately, checking and knowing your liver test results is one of the simplest and most science-backed steps you can take to protect your health, and the hacks in Chapter 2 can help you with this step. The good news is that early detection matters. A simple blood test, and sometimes an ultrasound, can catch issues long before symptoms appear. If you have one or more risk factors, ask your healthcare provider about liver screening. Knowledge is power—by knowing your risks, you can take steps to prevent progression and keep your liver healthy for decades to come.

In addition to early detection there are many other steps you can take to improve your liver health. Chapter 3 will guide you through the foods you can eat to boost your liver's wellness, as well as provide tips for healthy, mindful eating. The hacks in Chapter 4 will show you how exercise (no matter how minimal) will help your liver heal and repair itself, as well as take some of the burden off your liver by helping to push toxins out of your body. Chapter 5 will address being smart about all those liver "health" supplements you see on the market: Are they worth your time and money, and do they actually do anything beneficial for your liver? This chapter will also cover how to cut toxins and harmful additives from your diet. Lastly, Chapter 6 will show you that the smallest things—even sleeping—can improve the health of your liver. Rest and self-care practices can help rebuild your liver health, and the hacks in this chapter will show you how.

Chapter 2

TEST, TRACK, AND TAKE CHARGE

The liver is often a silent sufferer, and many liver conditions and diseases can be asymptomatic for years. In fact, MASLD (previously called fatty liver disease), hepatitis, and autoimmune liver disease can harm the liver for years without any warning signs, and by the time symptoms appear, the damage can be severe. Fortunately, there are many metrics you can track now to monitor the health of your liver, and this chapter will help you understand what they are and what they measure. Many can be detected with simple blood tests, and others are physical markers you can monitor on your own, such as your blood pressure and waist-to-hip ratio. This chapter will help you better understand these tests and empower you to make informed decisions about your care.

1

KNOW THE SIGNS OF A LIVER PROBLEM

Liver disease is usually silent, often not giving clues that something is brewing, which makes it even more important that you know the signs of a liver problem and act fast when those signs show up. When many people think of liver disease, they visualize someone who may appear jaundiced (yellowing of the skin), but that is most often a sign of severe liver inflammation and possible liver failure, not a common clue to a liver *problem*.

Possible clues that you may have a problem with your liver health may include fatigue, weakness, or aches on the right side of your body. Other concerning clues could include dark urine, pale stools, yellowing of the eyes or skin, easy bruising or bleeding, or distension of the abdomen. People may also have reduced appetite, nausea, or itchy skin. Serious warning signs in advanced liver disease could further include confusion, brain fog, or even coma.

The acronym "JAUNDICE" may help you remember the common symptoms:

- **J** = jaundice
- **A** = appetite loss
- **U** = urine darkening
- **N** = nausea or vomiting
- **D** = distended belly
- **I** = itchy skin
- **C** = confusion/brain fog
- **E** = easy bruising/bleeding

Don't wait until your symptoms progress to seek help. If you are experiencing any of the previous symptoms, seek medical attention or go to an emergency room.

2

TRACK YOUR ALT

Alanine aminotransferase (ALT) is a liver enzyme that lives inside your liver cells. Think of it as a "marker" of liver cell health. When your liver cells are injured or stressed—whether from too much fat, alcohol, medications, or viruses—they leak ALT into your blood where it doesn't belong. A simple blood test can show this rise and give you the impetus to take action.

A normal ALT is usually under 30 units/L (units per liter) for men and under 20 units/L for women, though ranges may vary by lab. If you have risk factors, such as type 2 diabetes, obesity, high cholesterol, regular alcohol intake, or a family history of liver disease, it is even more important that you check your ALT levels regularly. In terms of results, remember that mild elevations of ALT don't always mean serious disease, but they are a signal for you to look deeper. Conversely, a normal ALT does not necessarily mean your liver is completely healthy. If you have persistently high ALT levels, it suggests that you have ongoing liver stress that should not be ignored.

Next, use your ALT level as feedback. If it is high, talk to your doctor, adjust your lifestyle, and repeat the test in 3–6 months. You can lower your ALT through weight loss, exercise, balanced eating, and avoiding excess alcohol, and all these actions will improve your liver function and lower your long-term risk.

Discovering your ALT level is simple, inexpensive, and a powerful tool in your health journey. Know your number, track it over time, and use it as a tool to keep your liver strong.

3

USE AST AS YOUR GUIDE

Aspartate aminotransferase (AST) is another enzyme found in your liver cells, but it is also in muscle cells, heart muscle cells, and kidney cells. Like ALT (see previous entry), it leaks into the bloodstream when your cells are damaged. Because AST comes from more than just the liver, it is less specific than ALT, but it still plays a key role in understanding your liver health.

A normal AST is usually under 30 units/L for men and under 20 units/L for women, though this can vary by lab. You should be especially diligent about checking your AST if you have risks for liver disease, such as type 2 diabetes, obesity, alcohol use, viral hepatitis, or family history of liver disease. A high AST can be a signal of liver inflammation, but AST levels can also rise after muscle injury, such as from heavy exercise or heart problems.

Always look at your AST levels together with your ALT levels, as doctors often use the AST/ALT ratio to learn more about liver health. A ratio above 2 is often linked to alcohol injury, while a different pattern may suggest fatty liver or other causes.

Use AST as your guide. If it is elevated, discuss it with your doctor, check other liver tests, and make lifestyle changes.

4

CHECK YOUR ALP LEVELS

Alkaline phosphatase (ALP) is an enzyme found in your liver, bile ducts, intestinal tract, and bones. In the liver, low ALP levels signify the healthy flow of bile (the fluid that digests fats) through the bile ducts. When these ducts become blocked or inflamed, ALP levels in your blood often rise. If you are monitoring your ALP levels, you will have advanced notice that something is off with your liver's health.

Be sure to monitor your ALP levels if you have risk factors such as gallstones, heavy alcohol use, fatty liver disease, or unexplained bone pain. A normal ALP usually falls between 30 and 120 units/L, though exact ranges vary by lab and age. Also keep in mind that children and teens have higher ALP because their bones are still growing, and pregnant women have high levels of ALP, as it is also produced by the placenta.

A high ALP level may suggest liver or bile duct disease, but it can also point to bone conditions, so doctors will need to look at patterns and other tests to tell where the problem is coming from. This explains why doctors often pair ALP with other tests, such as gamma-glutamyl transferase (GGT) (see the next entry) to confirm if the liver is the source. If your levels are elevated, further testing is advised, as this could signify fat in the liver or an autoimmune liver disease.

5

MONITOR LIFESTYLE IMPACT BY TESTING GGT

Gamma-glutamyl transferase (GGT) is an enzyme mainly found in your liver and bile ducts. It plays a role in moving amino acids through the body and helping your liver process toxins. When the liver or bile ducts are stressed by alcohol, fatty liver, medications, or blockage in the bile duct, GGT leaks into the blood and your levels rise. Having your GGT levels assessed will alert you to any potential problems, as elevated GGT levels often suggest early liver or bile duct injury, sometimes even before the symptoms appear.

A normal GGT for adults is usually under 40 units/L, though the exact range depends on the lab. Doctors often look at the levels of GGT together with ALP levels. If both are high, the problem is likely liver-related, but if only ALP is high, the problem may be bone-related. Also be aware that GGT is very sensitive to alcohol use, so levels can climb even with moderate drinking. You should check your GGT levels if you drink alcohol regularly, take multiple medications, or have risk factors like obesity, type 2 diabetes, or high cholesterol.

Elevations in your GGT levels are a wake-up call. If they are elevated, reduce your alcohol intake, review your medications with your doctor, improve your diet, and get more exercise. Lowering your GGT is linked to a lower risk of liver disease and better long-term liver health.

6

USE BILIRUBIN LEVELS AS YOUR GUIDEPOST

Bilirubin is a yellow substance your body makes when it breaks down old blood cells. Your liver normally processes bilirubin and sends it through your bile into your intestines. When the liver or bile ducts aren't working properly, or when too many red blood cells are being destroyed, bilirubin builds up in the blood and can cause a condition known as jaundice, in which the skin and eyes turn yellow.

A normal total bilirubin level for an adult is usually less than 20 μmol/L (micromoles per liter), though labs may vary. High bilirubin levels can mean several things:

- You have a liver injury.
- Your bile ducts are blocked.
- There is an increase in red blood cell breakdown.
- You have Gilbert's syndrome. This harmless condition can also cause mild elevations of bilirubin. This condition is more common in men, and those who have it are born with it.

It is important to check your bilirubin levels if you have unexplained fatigue, dark urine, pale stools, yellowing of the eyes, or risk factors like viral hepatitis, gallstones, or fatty liver disease.

Use your bilirubin levels as a guidepost. If they are elevated, your doctor will often order the full panel of liver enzymes and imaging to find the cause. Keeping bilirubin in a healthy range helps ensure your liver is processing waste efficiently.

7

CONTROL YOUR BLOOD SUGAR

Having high blood sugar puts your liver at serious risk. High blood sugar and insulin resistance cause fat to build up in liver cells. The resulting condition, called metabolic dysfunction–associated steatotic liver disease (MASLD), is one of the most common complications of type 2 diabetes, and they often coexist.

You should recognize that extra sugar in your blood gets turned into fat and is stored in the liver. Over time, this fat triggers inflammation and scarring. Left unchecked, it can progress to cirrhosis and even liver cancer. Additionally, diabetes also worsens cholesterol and blood pressure, creating a cycle that accelerates liver injury and risks for cardiovascular disease.

Regular monitoring is key! If you have type 2 diabetes, you need to check your numbers. Ask your doctor to test your liver enzymes (ALT, AST, ALP, GGT, bilirubin), calculate a FIB-4 index (see entry later in this chapter), and perform an abdominal ultrasound. Many people with normal blood work may still have silent liver disease, so regular checking is important.

If your blood sugar is high, you need to get it under control with diet, exercise, and medications if needed. Losing 5–7 percent of your body weight has been shown to reduce liver fat and will improve your blood sugar. Exercise also improves insulin sensitivity and helps the liver burn off stored fat. If you keep your blood sugar levels steady, your liver will stay stronger, longer.

8

BE MINDFUL OF ALCOHOL CONSUMPTION

Each time you drink, your liver works to break down the alcohol. In the process, toxic by-products form that injure liver cells, trigger inflammation, and encourage toxic fat buildup. Over time, this repeated stress can lead to alcohol-related liver disease. Because of this, it is important that you are aware of not just how much alcohol you consume, but also the ways you can work to reduce the effects of alcohol on your liver and improve your health. Here are some things you can do:

- **Recognize the stages.** In the beginning, too much alcohol consumption causes fatty liver, which is often silent and without symptoms. However, if you continue to drink, inflammation develops (called alcohol hepatitis). If this injury continues, scar tissue begins to replace healthy cells, leading to cirrhosis. At this stage, the liver may be permanently damaged.
- **Look honestly at your intake.** Even moderate drinking can cause harm if it's regular. More than two drinks a day for men or one drink a day for women increases your risk, and binge drinking adds extra damage. Take an honest look at how much you drink and how frequently you drink, and work on reducing it if necessary.
- **Act to protect yourself.** Cut back on alcohol, set alcohol-free days each week, or quit entirely if your liver tests are abnormal. Also, don't forget to protect your liver with balanced eating, hydration, and medical checkups.

By reducing your alcohol intake now, you give your liver the chance to heal, lower inflammation, and prevent irreversible liver disease.

9

PROTECT AGAINST HEPATITIS B & C

Hepatitis B and C are viruses that directly attack your liver. They infect liver cells, trigger chronic inflammation, and silently cause injury over years. This ongoing stress leads to scarring (fibrosis) and cirrhosis, and raises your risk of liver cancer. To protect yourself from these viruses, take these steps:

- **Recognize the risks.** Hepatitis B spreads through blood and body fluids, unprotected sex, shared needles, or from mother to child at birth. Hepatitis C spreads mainly through blood exposure, such as shared needles, unsafe medical equipment, or transfusions before the early 1990s.
- **Check your status.** Both infections can be detected if liver enzymes are elevated; however, in many people, liver enzymes will be normal and the only way to find out is to get tested specifically for these viruses. A simple blood test tells you if you have been exposed, are infected, or are immune (for hepatitis B). For hepatitis C, blood tests, and sometimes viral load checks, confirm infection. If you test positive, doctors will monitor your liver enzymes and viral levels, and they may order imaging or special scans to assess damage.
- **Prevention is key!** Get vaccinated against hepatitis B if you are not protected. For hepatitis C, there is no vaccination yet; however, effective antiviral pills can cure the infection in almost everyone. For both viruses, treatment reduces the risk of cirrhosis, liver failure, and cancer.

Protect your liver. By knowing your status and seeking treatment, you can stop silent damage, prevent scarring, and keep your liver strong for life.

10

KNOW YOUR GENETIC HISTORY

Your genes and family history play a powerful role in liver health. If close relatives have had liver disease, such as fatty liver, cirrhosis, hepatitis, or liver cancer, you may carry a higher risk. Some conditions, like hemochromatosis (iron overload), Wilson's disease (copper buildup), celiac disease, and autoimmune liver disease, carry higher risks of being inherited. Additionally, gene variants (such as PNPLA3) that accelerate fat buildup and fibrosis progression have been identified in Hispanic and Latino populations. East and South Asians face a risk of aggressive liver disease at body weights that wouldn't raise a red flag on a standard BMI chart. In contrast, African Americans carry a protective version of the same gene despite higher rates of obesity and type 2 diabetes. But, even when the disease itself isn't inherited, shared lifestyle habits, like diet, alcohol use, or obesity, can increase risk within families.

Recognize that your family history is more than a detail—it is a warning sign. If liver problems run in your family, you may develop disease earlier or progress more quickly than someone without those risks. Ask your relatives if they have had liver disease, needed a transplant, or had unexplained cirrhosis or liver cancer. Then share this information with your doctor. They may recommend earlier screening with blood tests, ultrasounds, or genetic testing. In addition, you should try to maintain a healthy weight, limit alcohol, and get vaccinated against hepatitis A and B. If your family history suggests inherited conditions, follow through with recommended monitoring or preventative treatment.

11

TRACK YOUR WAISTLINE

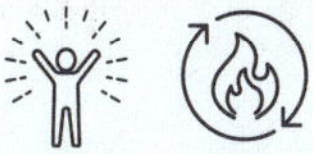

An enlarging waistline directly stresses your liver. When you carry too much fat, especially around the belly, your liver begins storing fat inside its own cells. This buildup used to be referred to as fatty liver disease but has been reclassified as MASLD: metabolic dysfunction–associated steatotic liver disease.

Recognize that fat in the liver is not harmless. It triggers inflammation, scarring, and eventually fibrosis. Over time, this scarring can progress to cirrhosis, where the liver becomes stiff and loses its ability to function efficiently. Obesity also fuels insulin resistance, high cholesterol, and high blood pressure, each one accelerating liver injury.

Check your waist size by measuring around the level of your belly button. Even if your blood work looks normal, silent fat accumulation may already be happening. Don't wait for lab results to tell you trouble is coming. Use this quick check as your early warning system to protect your liver and overall metabolic health.

GENDER	**WAIST** circumference in centimeters	**WAIST** circumference in inches	**RISK**
Men	Less than 94	Less than 37	Low
	94–102	37–40	Increased
	Greater than 102	Greater than 40	High
Women	Less than 80	Less than 31½	Low
	80–88	31½–35	Increased
	Greater than 88	Greater than 35	High

12

CALCULATE YOUR WAIST-TO-HIP RATIO

As weight is a key factor in stress on your liver, it's important to know where you stand. Not too long ago, doctors would use your body mass index (BMI) as a way of determining if your weight was in a healthy range. To find your BMI, you take your weight in kilograms and divide it by your height in meters squared. (Luckily there are several free online calculators if math isn't your thing.) A BMI between 18.5 and 24.9 is the lower end for metabolic and liver risk. A BMI below 18.5 is underweight and carries other risks. A BMI of 25–29.9 is overweight, a BMI of 30–34.9 is obese class I, a BMI of 35–39.9 is obese class II, and a BMI greater than 40 is obese class III. However, a very important limitation of BMI is that it does not separate muscle from fat stores, so an athlete may score "high" even if healthy. Additionally, there are ethnic variations to BMI ranges. Given these limitations, most healthcare providers no longer focus on BMI but rather on waist-to-hip ratio.

Your waist-to-hip ratio is a simple measurement anyone can do with a measuring tape—no fancy calculators are needed! Take your measuring tape and measure around your waist; write it down. Take another measurement around the widest part of your hips and write that down. Divide your waist measurement by your hip measurement, and if your waist is a higher value than your hips, this signifies higher cardiovascular risk and tends to match an "apple" shape versus a "pear" shape, which is lower risk. More accurate ratios are:

- Men: < 0.9 is low risk; > 0.9 is higher risk (apple shape)
- Women: < 0.85 is low risk; > 0.85 is higher risk (apple shape)

13

TRACK YOUR BLOOD PRESSURE OFTEN

The cause-effect relationship between high blood pressure (or hypertension) and fatty liver disease is unclear. Does the excess fat in your liver cause high blood pressure, or does high blood pressure cause fatty liver disease? The issue isn't obvious, but as these conditions often coexist, high blood pressure should be a red flag for you in terms of your liver's health. Tracking your blood pressure is one way you can monitor both your liver and cardiovascular health.

A healthy or normal blood pressure is 120/80, unless your clinician has set a different target for you. If your blood pressure is creeping upward, you need to trim your salt intake, move your body more, sleep 7–9 hours a night, and follow your medication plan.

To track your blood pressure at home, get an at-home blood pressure measuring kit, then measure your pressure at the same time each morning, usually after peeing and before you have coffee or take any pills. You should sit and rest for 5 minutes before you test, keeping your feet flat and back supported and keeping your arm on a table at heart level. Use an automated, validated upper-arm cuff and avoid wrist monitors if possible. Take two readings, 1 minute apart, and record the lower value.

Log your results in your phone or a notebook, and note your alcohol and salt intakes, as well as your sleep and stress patterns. Bring your log to healthcare visits and discuss trends with your doctor. Small steps add up over time, so measure, log, adjust, repeat. It's one easy task you can do each day to guard your liver health.

14

CHECK YOUR BLOOD SUGAR ROUTINELY

The repeated glucose spikes that come with high blood sugar drive insulin resistance and convert excess energy to fat, worsening MASLD and increasing the risk of liver inflammation and fibrosis. You need to flatten these spikes to lighten your liver's load and improve your liver and heart health.

Make awareness of your blood sugar a daily routine if you are prediabetic or have type 2 diabetes mellitus. Check your fasting blood sugar on waking, before meals, and 2 hours after the first bite a few days each week. To test, first wash your hands, dry them well, and use a validated glucose meter or continuous glucose monitor (CGM). Prick the side of a fingertip, rotate sites, and change your lancets regularly. Take two readings if a number looks off, and log the lower value.

Also remember to log context, not just numbers. Note your meal composition, fiber, protein, timing, alcohol, sleep quality, stress, illness, and activity. Track averages and let your clinician set targets. Spot patterns such as rising morning fasting levels, big postmeal spikes, or bedtime lows. Note the impact of stress or physical exercise on your blood sugar.

If your readings are high, some science-backed ways to reduce blood sugar include front-loading your meals with fiber and protein, reducing refined carbohydrates and sugary drinks, and walking 10–15 minutes after meals. Also, don't forget to hydrate, sleep 7–9 hours a night, and take your medications as prescribed. Add in purposeful exercise to maintain and build your muscles if you are not already doing so.

15

MONITOR CHOLESTEROL LEVELS

The liver makes 80 percent of your body's cholesterol, building it from scratch from the carbohydrates, fats, and proteins you have consumed. Excess sugar and refined carbs are often bigger drivers of cholesterol than fatty foods because flooding the liver with sugar is like flooding it with raw building material. Two key types of cholesterol are high-density lipoprotein (HDL) (also known as good cholesterol) and low-density lipoprotein (LDL) (also known as bad cholesterol). The liver not only makes this cholesterol; it also clears it from your body.

Your cholesterol levels are predictive of liver and heart health. Get a baseline fasting lipid panel (total LDL-C, HDL-C, and triglycerides) and an ApoB blood test (measures the level of apolipoprotein B in the blood). You may need to repeat these tests as advised by your clinician. Track your numbers and note your weight, alcohol consumption, fiber intake, and exercise. All adults should also have an assessment of their lipoprotein(a) [LP(a)], which can be an indicator of genetic predisposition to cardiovascular disease and stroke.

If you need to bring down your cholesterol, meaning lower your LDL and raise your HDL, you need to make lifestyle changes. Raise soluble fiber intake (oats, psyllium, beans); replace refined carbs with whole foods; minimize sugar intake; prioritize omega-3-rich fish two times weekly; walk 30 minutes daily (more intense exercise may lead to more benefit); and lift weights two to three times per week. Also limit your alcohol intake, take statins or other prescriptions as advised by your doctor, and log any side effects and your lab dates. Monitor your cholesterol levels, track your progress, and protect your heart and liver together. If you have high Lp(a), discuss with your physician if additional medications are needed to reduce future cardiovascular risk.

16

KNOW YOUR FIB-4 INDEX

Liver fat is not a healthy sign. In fact, having excess fat in your liver is a strong indication that you may develop liver fibrosis. Almost 40 percent of the population is dealing with MASLD, and there is the risk that 30–40 percent of them may go on to develop liver fibrosis (MASH). If you have high triglycerides, high blood pressure, evidence of elevated blood sugar, or type 2 diabetes, then you are at higher risk of developing liver damage.

Unfortunately, blood tests are not always accurate, and liver blood tests can be normal while an ultrasound of the liver may show signs of liver fat. Therefore, your doctor may calculate your fibrosis-4 index (FIB-4) by entering your AST, ALT, platelet count, and age. The calculation will indicate whether you are at low, intermediate, or high risk of liver fibrosis and whether further testing is needed.

If you have any of the risk factors previously mentioned, have your FIB-4 calculated yearly to provide guidance on whether your liver disease is worsening. Assessment by a liver specialist may be warranted if you have an intermediate- or high-risk FIB-4, to rule out other possible liver diseases and provide treatment if advanced fibrosis is present. Subsequent liver fibrosis tests include Liver Elastography (FibroScan) and the Enhanced Liver Fibrosis (ELF) serum biomarker tests.

Knowing your FIB-4 index is just one more step in monitoring your liver health to help prevent further damage.

17

INVESTIGATE YOUR LOW PLATELETS

If you discover your platelet count is low, it is important that you investigate the possible causes, as a lower-than-normal platelet count is often an indicator of liver disease.

Platelets are just one of the body's mechanisms to help clot blood and are different from the clotting factors specifically manufactured by the liver. Your platelets are made in your bone marrow along with your red blood cells and are measured by your complete blood count (CBC), a routine and common blood test.

In terms of liver health, low platelets can signal an issue because if someone has advanced or chronic liver disease, they may have developed liver cirrhosis. As a consequence of this liver cirrhosis, the spleen (a triangular organ in the upper left side of the abdomen) may enlarge. When the spleen is enlarged, it can destroy the platelets made by your bone marrow. This will result in a lower-than-normal platelet count, which may indicate severe liver disease.

While it is true that other factors can cause a low platelet count with a normal, healthy liver—including a disease of the bone marrow or specific splenic disease—a low platelet count should always be evaluated to ensure advanced liver disease is not present.

18

USE A HEALTH TRACKER APP

A health tracker app is different from a fitness tracker app because a health tracker focuses on your broader, overall well-being and medical information, while a fitness tracker app focuses specifically on physical activity and performance. A health tracker app may also further track sleep, mood, and hydration, whereas a fitness app is more geared toward steps taken, workouts, and calorie burn from exercise. Both of these options provide low-cost participation in managing your healthcare, but the health tracker app can turn liver care into a daily system.

Using a health tracker app, you can build a custom dashboard that can log all your liver health needs, such as your blood pressure, weight, waist measurements, resting heart rate (RHR), sleep hours, hydration, fiber grams, protein servings, alcohol units, sugary drink intake, medications, herbal supplements, any symptoms, lab results, and more. There can even be a section for doctor appointment dates and vaccinations. You can also set reminders for medications, alcohol-free days, postmeal walks, and fasting labs.

To use the app effectively, create rules for yourself; for example, if your resting heart rate rises above 8 beats per minute (bpm) or your sleep falls below 6 hours, you need to take a recovery day.

Let fitness measure effort, let health tracking guide recovery, and liver outcomes will improve.

19

ASK FOR LIVER IMAGING/ ELASTOGRAPHY

If you have an enlarged waist, elevated weight, or are prediabetic or on treatment for type 2 diabetes, high blood pressure, or high cholesterol, then it is important that you ask your clinician for an abdominal ultrasound to check for visible fatty liver.

When you talk to your doctor about the possibility of having this liver imaging, bring a 4-week log of your weight, waist measurement, alcohol units, medications/supplements (including herbal), sleep, and exercise patterns. Talk to your doctor about why you feel the test is necessary, and use your log as backup. Then be sure your doctor uses clear wording when ordering the test. You want the test to assess for hepatic steatosis and biliary causes of liver enzyme elevation. If available, ask if they can add shear wave elastography (or FibroScan) to estimate liver stiffness and quantify fat.

If liver fat is present or your enzymes are elevated, request some of the previously mentioned labs—such as ALT, AST, GGT, ALP, bilirubin, and platelets—a FIB-4 fibrosis score (see entry in this chapter), and possibly an Enhanced Liver Fibrosis (ELF) test or FibroScan. Then set a 6–12-month follow-up. If stiffness scores are high, nodules appear, or enzymes stay up, ask for a gastroenterology, internal medicine, or hepatology referral. If you have known cirrhosis or hepatitis B, discuss having a liver ultrasound every 6 months for liver cancer surveillance, depending on your age, gender, fibrosis stage, or family history of liver cancer.

Then take action on your findings: Cut your alcohol intake, target losing 7–10 percent of your weight, and start an exercise program. Then reimage your liver to confirm improvement.

20

COMPARE YOUR ANNUAL TEST RESULTS

Treat your annual test results as a scoreboard for your liver improvement. Make your liver preventative care the best it can be by lining up the same labs every year and then reading the trends and not the one-off results. Book your testing the same month each year, at the same lab, ideally in the morning hours when you have fasted for 8–12 hours, have no alcohol in your system, and have had no hard workouts for 48–72 hours. When you level the playing field data-wise for your tests, the results can be a real measurable story of your progress.

Don't forget to sign up at your laboratory for an account to track your results—and if your lab doesn't offer this service, then keep a record yourself. Track your ALT, AST, GGT, ALP, bilirubin, platelets, Hb A1C, fasting lipids, triglycerides, TSH, iron studies, and viral hepatitis studies as per your clinician. Also, for the 2 weeks before each blood draw, log your weight, waist measurement, blood pressure, alcohol unit intake, any medications or supplements, sleep, and exercise. In addition, track your FIB-4 index if you have known MASLD.

But keeping track is only the first step in your liver health journey. Be sure to tie action to any trends you see, and if enzymes improve, keep up with your current plan. If there is no change or you are trending in the wrong direction, then honestly review your intake of alcohol and sugary drinks, along with your exercise frequency. If, after you implement your new changes, your numbers still don't improve, then further specialist assessment is advised.

21

TAKE CHARGE AT DOCTORS' VISITS

By taking charge at every doctor's visit, you can formulate a real plan with purpose for your liver and overall health rather than vague medical advice that you may not understand. Before each doctor visit, prepare a one-page brief with:

- Your top three goals (for example, lower ALT, cut liver fat, increase number of alcohol-free days).
- A 4-week log (tracking your weight, waist measurements, alcohol units, all medications or supplements [with doses], hours of sleep, and number of steps [or other exercise]).
- Any questions you may have.

Open the visit with a clear ask to know about your liver health and an action plan. Then discuss your baseline lab tests and viral screens. Next, discuss the following behaviors with your doctor, and treat them like prescriptions for your health:

- Target 7–10 percent weight loss if needed.
- Initiate 150–300 minutes per week of moderate activity.
- Perform two strength training sessions per week.
- Start after-meal walks.
- Set alcohol limits or consider abstinence.

Before you leave, repeat the plan (what, why, when) with your doctor and agree upon a monitoring interval, such as a retest in 3–6 months if needed. Then book your follow-up appointment before you leave that day. Remember, you are the best advocate for your health; don't let that opportunity slip away.

22

KNOW YOUR ALBUMIN LEVEL

Albumin is a blood protein made by the liver, and its measurement in the blood may indicate your liver's health and its ability to manufacture the essential building blocks of life. (One physical clue that your albumin may be low is swelling in your ankles to the point you can no longer see or feel the bony part of your ankle bone.) Since albumin is made by your liver, low values can signal chronic liver disease, inflammation, malnutrition, or even problems with the kidney or gut. The change in your albumin level over time matters more than a single number, so this is a level you will want to track and monitor.

With your next blood work panel, ask for your serum albumin to be measured, although it is often part of many liver panels. You'll want to see a normal adult range of 35–50 g/L (grams/liter) and confirm that with the lab's reference range.

If your levels are low, you need to protect and rebuild. Be sure to prioritize adequate protein intake daily per your clinician's guidance, with more protein intake advised if you have liver cirrhosis or ascites. Also try to distribute your protein intake evenly over meals, rather than lumping it all into one. Knowing and monitoring your albumin levels is an important step in the longevity of your liver.

23

SPOT SUGAR CRAVINGS QUICKLY

To improve your liver health, it's wise to track your hunger signals and catch your sugar cravings early so they don't sabotage your day or your liver. Here are some simple and effective ways to do this:

- Build meal anchors for yourself at consistent times to limit grazing (for example, breakfast at 7:00, lunch at 1:00, snack at 3:00, and so on).
- Avoid "naked" carbs (juice, candy, refined snacks) that spike insulin and promote liver fat.
- Have a plan in place for the hunger danger zone (2:00–5:00 p.m.). Prep high-protein snacks (such as Greek yogurt, nuts, eggs, and edamame) and avoid juice or soda.
- Keep sweets out of your sight and have savory, crunchy stand-ins handy (roasted chickpeas, carrots, and hummus).
- Before each meal/snack, rate your hunger on a scale from 0–10 (0 = not hungry, 10 = ravenous). The danger of waiting until you are ravenous to eat is that your body enters a "fight-or-flight" mode, which may lead you to eat too quickly, crave high-calorie/low-nutrient foods, and eat past the point of fullness. If you're already at an 8–10, then drink water first (to help fill your stomach) and wait 10–15 minutes. Then choose a protein and a fiber-rich snack to stabilize glucose and reduce liver fat drivers.
- Brush your teeth or use a mint to "close the kitchen."
- Track sugar craving triggers (for example, less than 7 hours of sleep, stress, alcohol, skipped meals, and so on).

If your sugar cravings ever feel compulsive, you have mood shifts, or you engage in severe binging, ask your clinician for support.

24

KNOW YOUR CLOTTING FACTORS

The liver makes most of your body's clotting factors and natural blood thinners, such as protein C, protein S, and antithrombin. Changes in your clotting factors often reflect your liver's "synthetic" health. Ask for a clotting check with your next labs. This should include your prothrombin time (PT), international normalized ratio (INR), platelet count, and fibrinogen (plus liver enzymes). A rising INR or prolonged PT often appears first. Track your results and dates, and remember to focus on trends, not single numbers.

Next, protect your system. You'll want to:

- Avoid alcohol.
- Review any medications you take that raise bleeding risk, such as nonsteroidal anti-inflammatories (NSAIDs), aspirin, and some supplements like fish oil, gingko, and garlic.
- Discuss any prescription blood thinners (warfarin, direct oral anticoagulants [DOACs]) with your clinician and never stop or start those medications on your own.

Finally, know the signals of clotting problems. Seek urgent care for black, tarry stools; vomiting blood; bright red rectal bleeding; severe nose/gum bleeds; large spontaneous bruises; or oozing. Before you have any dental work or procedures, share your liver history, latest INR/platelets, and medication list so a plan is in place to minimize your bleeding risk.

25

CHECK YOUR URINE COLOR

The color of your urine is often your fastest hydration and liver check. You should aim for a pale-straw color to light yellow for most of the day. Dark yellow to amber often means you are dehydrated. If you see this, drink water and check again in a few hours. You should check your urine color every morning and again midafternoon. If your urine stays dark despite good liquid intake, you should ask your doctor or clinician for liver and urine tests.

Some urine colors to be wary of:

- Tea-colored/brown urine in combination with pale, clay-colored stools, itching, fatigue, right upper abdominal discomfort, or yellow eyes/skin can be a signal of bilirubin buildup from cholestasis or hepatitis, and you should seek urgent care.
- Reddish or pink urine that is not a result of beets, berries, or a hard workout may be a sign of blood in the urine.
- Orange urine can come from dehydration, bile duct disease, or medications such as rifampin.
- Neon yellow urine is usually from B vitamins.
- Green/blue urine may be from dyes or medications.
- Persistently foamy urine can reflect protein loss, and this will warrant a urinalysis.

Support your liver by keeping hydrated, eating water-rich foods, and limiting alcohol and caffeine. In addition, if you're sweating heavily, remember to replace electrolytes. Note that fever, vomiting, and diarrhea can all darken urine, so treat the cause of those aliments and then recheck your urine color.

26

LOOK AT YOUR POOP

For a comprehensive liver (and gut health) check, make a 10-second bathroom check part of your liver care routine. Note the color, shape, and sheen of your stool. Use the Bristol Stool Chart to help you decipher what you see, keeping in mind that Bristol types 3–4 are the ideal.

BRISTOL STOOL CHART TYPE	APPEARANCE	SUGGESTIVE OF
Type 1	Separate hard lumps, like nuts	Constipation
Type 2	Sausage-shaped but lumpy	Constipation
Type 3	Sausage with cracks on surface	Normal
Type 4	Smooth, soft, snakelike	Normal
Type 5	Soft blobs with clear edges	Low fiber/borderline loose
Type 6	Fluffy pieces with ragged edges; mushy	Mild diarrhea
Type 7	Watery, no solid pieces	Severe diarrhea

STOOL COLOR	WHAT IT MAY INDICATE
Pale, clay, puttylike	Impaired bile flow
Greasy, foul, floating	Fat malabsorption
Bright red	Lower gut bleeding, beets
Black, tarry	Upper gut bleeding
Greenish	Fast transit or leafy foods
Dark but not tarry	May reflect intake of iron or bismuth

One odd stool is common, but persistent change matters. Track your poop for a week and reflect on what you ate and drank during this time; be sure to factor in your sleep and hydration as well.

27

BUILD YOUR OWN HEALTH STORY

Because liver issues can often be overwhelming, it's important for you to build a one-page liver health snapshot and bring it with you to every doctor visit. Having all your information in one centralized document will help you keep organized about your health and ensure that any new medical professional can get a quick overview of your history and issues. Here are some items you should list on your story:

- Any diagnoses and the dates of diagnosis.
- Any procedures you have had and the dates.
- Key medical contacts.
- Core lab tests you've had and your tracking that shows trends.
- Any imaging and biopsy results with dates.
- Your medication list with doses, dose changes, timing, and start dates. Be sure to include a list for over-the-counter medications, herbal medications, and supplements.
- Your intake of alcohol and other substances, including recreational if using (cannabis, opiates, and so on).
- Your allergies and past reactions.
- Your vitals, such as blood pressure, weight, waist measurement, resting heart rate, daily steps, and exercise.
- Any vaccines you've gotten, the date you received them, and when they are next due.

After each doctor visit, write any new changes to your medical plan in your own words so it is understandable for you. Share updates with your healthcare team and trusted caregivers. Review your health story monthly, and revise it after all new results.

Chapter 3

FEED YOUR LIVER RIGHT

As the old saying goes, "You are what you eat," and the toxins found in the foods and beverages you consume will all have to pass through your digestive tract and liver. Your food and drink choices directly impact both how hard your liver will have to work and if your liver will have enough of the essential nutrients needed for optimal function. It is also essential to appreciate the importance of your gut microbiome—those trillions of bacteria living in your gut are dynamic, adapting and responding to your environment and playing a big role in your systemic (and even mental) health. Diet and lifestyle changes can alter the gut microbiome in as little as 5 days! This chapter will teach you the foods and beverages that harm your liver as well as those that will help heal your liver. You'll find practical approaches and lots of variety so you can make the food changes that are realistic and sustainable for your everyday life.

28

WRITE DOWN YOUR DAILY BEVERAGES

Hydration is a key marker in improving your liver's health, but so many of us forget to drink during the day or drink beverages that harm rather than help our livers. Both alcoholic and sugary drinks drive liver fat, inflammation, and injury, and repeated hits raise triglycerides, blood pressure, and insulin resistance. The first step in improving is to track the drinks you are consuming, both for your own knowledge and as a metric to share with your doctor.

Log every beverage you consume for 7 days. This includes alcohol, juice, sodas, energy drinks, fancy coffees, and mocktails. Record the time you drank it; the type; the volume; and, for alcohol, the alcohol by volume (ABV) percentage. For example:

- 12 ounces beer = 5 percent
- 5 ounces wine = 12 percent
- 1½ ounces spirit = 40 percent

Add quick tags to your log, such as "with dinner," "stress," "social," or "after workout," to help you remember the circumstances surrounding your intake. Also, note your sleep quality and mood the next morning.

Next, total your daily and weekly counts. Circle any patterns you see. Then discuss your log and set a plan with your doctor.

Use your log to cut total doses, shrink portions, and avoid late-night consumption to protect your sleep. Let cleaner choices lighten your liver's load!

29

REDUCE SUGARY BEVERAGES

Reducing the number of sugary drinks you consume improves your blood sugar levels, which helps protect your liver from developing fatty liver and insulin resistance. Tracking your intake will make you more aware of both your sugar consumption and your calorie consumption.

For 7 days, write down every sweetened beverage you drink. In your log, record the time consumed, the brand, the size of the drink and any add-ins (syrups, sweeteners, cream), the total calories, and the total sugar in grams. Use the following guidelines to honestly assess your beverages:

- **Measure, don't guess.** Learn your usual glass size by pouring into a measuring cup once. For takeout, use the posted size; if the drink is iced, assume half the cup is ice unless noted.
- **Read the label for total sugar grams.** If your beverage doesn't have a label, look up the chain's nutrition page or choose a close match.

At the end of the week, review your log. Find your top three sugar sources and devise a swap for each. Here are some ways to reduce the number of sugary drinks you consume:

- Choose smaller sizes.
- Choose unsweetened versions.
- Order the drink 25–50 percent sweet, as the syrups are often dispensed in pumps where amount can be controlled.

Aim to consume these drinks less over time, and soon they will become unpalatable as your taste buds adjust. Your liver and overall metabolic health will benefit.

30

KEEP A FOOD JOURNAL

To be more successful in reaching your goals to improve liver health, commit to keeping a 2-week food journal. The act of journaling your food will make you more conscious of what you are putting into your body and the quality of foods you consume.

Your journal can take any form you choose; in fact, the more comfortable you are with your journaling method, the more likely you are to use it. You can use the Notes app, Google Sheets, or even a small notebook for your journal. In your journal, create a table to record the time you ate, your hunger score (1–10), the cooking method, any drinks, and any added sugars. Note the number of vegetables, proteins, refined carbohydrates, and your daily water intake. Track daily totals and even take photos of your meals and snacks to help with tracking and accountability.

Each day calculate if you have reached the recommended targets of:

- 30–38 grams of fiber per day
- 1.2–1.6 grams per kilogram of protein per day (roughly 25–30 grams per meal)

Achieving these goals can be hard, but meal prepping—by making meals in bulk and dividing them up into preportioned servings—can help you feel more prepared and be more successful in reaching your goals to improve liver health.

31

IMPROVE YOUR FIBER INTAKE

Fiber is a critical piece in protecting your liver health. A diet high in fiber stabilizes insulin, lowers LDL, makes you feel full or satiated, feeds the gut microbes that make anti-inflammatory short-chain fatty acids (SCFAs), and reduces the visceral fat that drives fatty liver and MASLD. For these reasons, it is important to be aware of your fiber intake. You should aim for 25–35 grams per day, which is roughly 7–10 grams per meal.

In your food journal (see previous entry) you'll want to write "fiber" beside each meal and jot the grams of fiber contained in that meal so you can easily see what your daily intake is. You can also make a list of some high-fiber foods you wish to incorporate into your diet. Here are a few good examples:

- 1 tablespoon chia/flax = 5 grams fiber
- ½ cup beans = 7–9 grams (depending on type)
- 1 cup raspberries = 8 grams
- 1 medium pear or apple = 5 grams
- 1 cup cooked broccoli = 5 grams
- ½ cup cooked oats/barley/quinoa = 4–6 grams
- 2 slices whole-grain bread = 5–8 grams

Increase your fiber intake gradually, adding about 5 grams a day each week until your target goal is reached, and don't forget to drink plenty of water to reduce gas. Your microbiome will thank you, and your gut and heart will too!

32

HYDRATE DAILY

In order to improve the health of your liver, you need to stay hydrated. Fluid intake influences energy, appetite, and liver workload, so you need to treat your hydration needs as if they were a prescription for your health.

Make your hydration an automatic part of your day. Keep a marked bottle of water on your desk and drink 16 ounces (approximately 500 milliliters) on waking, 12–16 ounces (approximately 300–500 milliliters) with or after each meal, and small sips hourly. Pair each caffeinated drink you consume with a glass of water and log all your alcohol separately as that is not considered hydration. For proper hydration, you should favor water, unsweetened tea, or sparkling water and avoid sugar-sweetened beverages. Don't forget to add in some hydrating foods, such as citrus, cucumber, and low-sodium broth-based soups as well.

Watch for safety flags such as rapid weight gain, leg swelling, shortness of breath, confusion, or persistent dark urine or reduced urination. If these issues occur, contact your clinician. If you have heart, kidney, or advanced liver disease (ascites), use the self-targets given to you by your doctor.

33

MAKE WATER YOUR FIRST DRINK OF THE DAY

When you consistently make water your first drink of the day, this small, repeated action compounds into steadier energy, gentler digestion, and a happier liver.

Even before you have your morning coffee, tea, juice, or food, pour yourself 1–2 cups (approximately 300–500 milliliters) of water upon waking and sip it steadily. This morning water rehydrates your overnight losses so your liver and kidneys can remove nutrients and waste efficiently and do what they were designed to do. Keeping hydrated with water also supports bile production and smoother digestion.

Drinking water often curbs morning cravings, and since thirst often masquerades as hunger, starting your morning with water reduces cravings for impulsive high-sugar and high-calorie foods that can stress your liver. In addition, drinking your water 10–15 minutes before you drink any form of caffeine can lessen the jitters and dehydration that coffee alone can cause.

Drinking plain, cool or room-temperature water is ideal. Try keeping reusable bottles accessible—one by your bed and one by your desk. Repeat the "water first" rule before each meal as well (a half cup is enough) to pace your eating and reduce your intake of sugary beverages. Add a squeeze of citrus to your water if you need flavor, but skip adding in any sweeteners. If you have heart, kidney, or liver failure, follow your clinician's guidance to prevent overhydration in special circumstances.

34

ADD CITRUS TO ENHANCE HYDRATION

You know already that you need to drink more water to improve your liver's well-being. But what if drinking plain water bores you? Adding flavor with natural citrus may be the winning change you need. Adding citrus, like a squeeze of orange, lime, or lemon, can make a difference in improving your hydration goals—and your liver's health.

Squeeze 1/4 to 1/2 of a fresh lemon into 1 to 2 cups of water and drink it first thing in the morning and before each meal. You can also try making lemon ice cubes and keep them in the freezer for busy mornings.

Adding citrus to your water not only helps make it more palatable, but it also delivers vitamin C to support collagen, immunity, and normal antioxidant defenses. In addition, the citrus polyphenols in the pulp and zest help counter everyday oxidative stress, and the citric acid boosts urinary citrate and may lower the risk of kidney stones—good news for your overall health.

Upgrade your hydration with citrus and enjoy the clean, bright taste so you can reach for water instead of sugary drinks that burden the liver. Add a pinch of pulp or a thin, well-washed strip of zest for extra aroma, and be sure to skip the sugars and artificial sweeteners. If you have acid reflux, mouth sores, or enamel sensitivity, go lighter on the citrus or use plain water. Otherwise, enjoy this tiny, tasty upgrade to improve your hydration and your liver health!

35

SIP ON BROTH

Bone broth and mineral-rich broths are underrated allies for your liver health. Your liver works nonstop to detoxify, regulate metabolism, and support immune balance, and it needs the right building blocks to do that efficiently. Broth provides easily absorbed amino acids such as glycine, proline, and glutamine that support liver detox pathways and help make a healthy gut. And when you have a healthier gut, there are fewer toxins and inflammatory by-products reaching the liver.

Some specific ways broth is beneficial for your body include:

- The glycine broth provides plays a direct role in phase 2 liver detoxification, where the liver packages toxins so they can be safely excreted. In addition, adequate glycine availability may reduce oxidative stress and inflammation in liver cells.
- Broth may also support bile flow, which is needed for fat digestion and toxin elimination.
- Broth is naturally hydrating and rich in electrolytes such as sodium, potassium, and magnesium, all key for maintaining blood volume and cellular function, particularly if you exercise, fast, or sweat frequently.
- Unlike sugary drinks or processed soups, a clean homemade or low-additive broth avoids fructose, preservatives, and inflammatory oils that burden the liver.

For best results, you should sip broth between meals or in the evening as a calming ritual. Choose slow-simmered bone broth or vegetable broth with minimal ingredients. Simple, nourishing, and restorative, broth provides the support your liver needs.

36

TRY GREEN TEA

Green tea contains catechins that may help to improve liver fat, support a healthy weight, and help with lipid management. Try to swap one sugary drink a day for a mug of unsweetened green tea to improve your liver health. Then make it a goal to aim for 2–3 cups daily to nudge your metabolism and reduce liver fat drivers from excess sugar.

Start by brewing your green tea correctly: Heat your water to hot but not boiling (78°F–85°F), add your tea bag (or loose leaves) and allow it to steep 2–3 minutes, then remove the bag or strain the leaves to avoid bitterness. (Using boiling water can scorch the delicate catechins and amino acids in green tea, particularly L-theanine.) You can also squeeze in some fresh lemon juice to brighten the flavor and help protect the catechins. Prefer iced tea? Try cold brew by adding 1–2 teaspoons loose leaves to 250–300 milliliters of cold water and allowing it to steep in the refrigerator for 6–8 hours.

You can also use green tea as a hunger brake. When a craving hits, make your green tea first before you reach for a snack, and sip it slowly and mindfully. This calming ritual plus the warm fluid often curbs snack impulses. You can also try matcha (a premium Japanese green tea) when you want a little more focus (use 1/2 to 1 teaspoon whisked with hot water) and choose decaf varieties after noon if caffeine keeps you up.

For safety, avoid high-dose green tea extract pills. If you're pregnant, iron deficient, or take medications (especially warfarin, beta-blockers, or statins), check with your doctor and be sure to drink your tea at least an hour away from when you take your iron supplements to avoid inadvertently binding the iron, making it ineffective.

37

SNACK ON NUTS

Swap your usual chips, candy, or pastries for a small handful (about 30 grams) of nuts once or twice a day. This swap will give you healthy fats, plant protein, and fiber that helps control appetite, smooths blood sugar swings, and reduces late-night binge calories that drive fat storage in the liver. In addition, the monounsaturated and polyunsaturated fats in nuts will help improve your LDL/HDL balance, which supports your metabolic health. Better metabolic health means less visceral fat and less liver fat. This helps reduce the liver's fat-handling burden and supports healthier ALT and AST over time.

When choosing your nuts, go for unsalted nuts such as almonds, walnuts, pistachios, pecans, hazelnuts, or peanuts. Pair those nuts with fruit or Greek yogurt to add fiber and volume without the sugar spikes. You could also sprinkle chopped walnuts on oatmeal and salads or consider spreading 1 tablespoon of nut butter on apple slices or whole-grain toast.

Use nuts to replace your snacks, not add additional snacks. Trade your usual muffin for nuts and berries. Trade those nachos for pistachios and sliced cucumber. Trade that milk chocolate snack for two squares of dark chocolate and crushed walnuts. Watch your serving sizes and remember to eat the nuts slowly, not mindlessly, so that you don't overeat.

You can also try roasting your own nuts by toasting them at 300°F (150°C) for 10–12 minutes to brighten their flavor, and then store any extras in the freezer to protect their healthy, delicate oils. Toss your smoked nuts with chili powder, smoked paprika, or a pinch of sea salt, plus lemon zest for even more flavor.

38

EAT FISH WEEKLY

Aim to have fish two times per week, prioritizing fatty fishes such as salmon, sardines, mackerel, trout, and herring. Not only will this swap be beneficial to your liver because it will replace the red or processed meats you usually eat, but the EPA/DHA omega-3s in fish will help to lower triglycerides, calm liver inflammation, and support insulin sensitivity, which are the key levers for reducing liver fat.

Set a weekly seafood night and stock quick options such as canned salmon, light tuna, or sardines for when you are short on time. Keep cooking simple by baking, grilling, or poaching your fish, and be sure to avoid deep-frying your seafood. Season the fish with lemon, garlic, herbs, and a drizzle of olive oil for a liver-friendly dish, and pair it with fiber-rich sides (like roasted vegetables, beans, or whole grains) to help carry cholesterol and bile acids out of the body.

When choosing your fish, look for low-mercury species and limit any high-mercury fish, such as shark, swordfish, king mackerel, tilefish, and bigeye tuna. If you're pregnant or breastfeeding, choose low-mercury options and cap your albacore tuna intake at one serving per week. Keep portions palm-sized (about 100–150 grams cooked) and chill any leftovers within 2 hours.

Don't eat fish? Consider an algae-based EPA/DHA supplement (1–2 grams/day) after checking first with your clinician. If you use anticoagulants or plan to take high-dose fish oil, confirm their safety with your care team.

39

FILL YOURSELF WITH FIBER

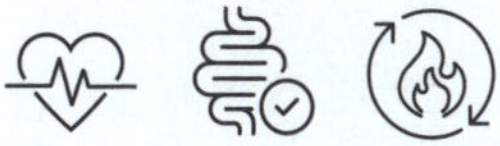

Fiber is your liver's friend, not only helping to calm inflammation and reduce liver fat, but aiding digestion and elimination as well. Try soluble fiber (oats, barley, psyllium, beans) to bind bile acids and LDL cholesterol, nudging your body to pull more cholesterol from circulation and easing the liver workload. Use insoluble fiber (bran, vegetable skins, whole grains) to keep your bowel habits regular so waste leaves your body promptly. Fiber will also feed your gut microbes with more short-chain fatty acids, which means better insulin sensitivity, which will calm inflammation and liver fat.

Add more fiber to your diet, starting with 10–15 grams the first week, then building up to 30 grams a day. Try these ideas:

- At breakfast, add oats, chia seeds, or ground flax or hemp seeds to your dishes.
- Swap white bread, rice, and pasta for whole-grain options, such as rye, barley, quinoa, or whole wheat.
- Add 1 cup of beans or lentils to soups, salads, tacos, or pasta dishes three to four times a week.
- Instead of chips, have a cup of berries or a pear or an apple with the skin on.
- Load your plate with vegetables at meals.
- Keep washed, cut produce at eye level in your refrigerator so you can reach for it first over packaged snacks.

Remember to drink 3–5 cups of water as you raise your fiber intake. If you have irritable bowel syndrome (IBS), favor soluble fiber and increase gradually.

40

COOK AT HOME

Foods of convenience have never been more accessible than they are now, but there is no doubt that cooking at home helps overall health and protects your liver and gut health. The benefits of cooking at home include that you control the ingredients, portions, and cooking methods so you can cut excess sugar, salt, and oils. In addition, by cooking at home you skip ultra-processed sauces and can instead season with garlic, spices, vinegar, and lemon, all of which keep flavor high and processed add-ons low.

Make cooking at home easy and stock a "liver pantry" that includes olive oil, canned tomatoes and beans, tuna/salmon, whole-wheat pasta, quinoa, oats, onions, ginger, garlic, frozen mixed vegetables, and spices. When you serve your meal, remember to fill your plate with two fists of vegetables, one palm of protein, one cupped hand of whole grains or beans, and a thumb-sized amount of oil.

To make cooking at home easier on busy nights, cook once and eat thrice by meal prepping. Cook one to two times per week and portion the meals into containers for easy dinners.

When you replace two restaurant meals per week with home cooking, both your liver and your wallet will benefit!

41

PICK FRESH FRUIT AND KEEP IN SEASON

Choose fresh fruit as your default sweet instead of the pastries, candy, and ultra-processed snacks that strain your metabolism and drive liver fat. Leverage fruit's natural fiber, water, potassium, and polyphenols to improve your liver health by taming blood sugar spikes, supporting bile flow, and calming low-grade inflammation. Aim for two or three servings of fruit daily, where one serving is the equivalent to one medium fruit, 1 cup of cut fruit, or 1 cup of berries.

To make it easy to choose fruit over other snacks, keep a bright fruit bowl on the counter and washed berries at eye level in the refrigerator. Pair your fruit with protein or fat like yogurt, cottage cheese, nuts, or peanut butter to feel fuller longer and to smooth glucose curves. Build simple default snacks that you always have on hand, such as an apple and almonds, an orange and yogurt, a banana and peanut/nut butter toast, or berries with oats.

Buy seasonal fruit for better taste and price. Choose whole fruit over juice, but if you do drink juice, try to limit it to ½ cup and dilute it with water. Here are some common fruits and the liver-healthy nutrients they provide:

FRUIT	NUTRIENT
Berries	Anthocyanins
Kiwis	Folate
Citrus	Vitamin C, hesperidin
Mangoes	Carotenoids
Grapes	Polyphenols
Apples/pears	Pectin

42

CHOOSE WHOLE GRAINS

Consuming whole grains as a regular part of your diet steadies blood sugar, lowers triglycerides and LDLs by binding bile acids, and feeds gut microbes that produce anti-inflammatory short-chain fatty acids. The result is reduced metabolic stress and reduced fat buildup in your liver—so eat those whole grains!

Try swapping any refined carbohydrates for whole grains at most of your meals. Aim for one to two servings of whole grains daily, and choose from grains like oats, barley, rye, whole wheat, brown or wild rice, quinoa, farro, and bulgur. At mealtimes, swap in brown rice, bulgur, or whole-wheat pasta for your typical carbs, and don't forget to add your two fist-sized portions of vegetables and one palm-sized protein portion to your plate. You can also make weekday mealtimes easier by batch-cooking a pot of grains on the weekend and freezing portions for later meals.

Also, shop smart and read those nutrition labels when shopping for whole grains, and aim for 3 grams of fiber per serving, less than 2 grams of sugar, and minimal additives. Start slow if you're new to fiber, and increase your daily intake slowly over a week. Also remember to drink more water and keep your portions consistent. If you have celiac disease, choose gluten-free options like oats (certified), quinoa, and brown rice.

43

COOK WITH OLIVE OIL

If liver health is on your mind, then extra-virgin olive oil (EVOO) should become your default fat. Harness its monounsaturated fats to improve LDL/HDL balance and triglycerides, which will ease the metabolic load that pushes fat into your liver. Leverage olive oil's polyphenols (like hydroxytyrosol and oleocanthal) to counter oxidative stress and quiet low-grade inflammation, which are two causes of liver injury.

Use olive oil to replace butter, shortening, and ultra-processed oils for frying. Dress salads, grain bowls, or beans and greens with 1–2 teaspoons of olive oil, or finish cooked vegetables, fish, or eggs with a drizzle, both for flavor and for better absorption of fat-soluble vitamins and carotenoids. Make quick vinaigrettes with it (3 parts EVOO, 1 part acid), and use EVOO in marinades to boost herb/spice antioxidants.

To make using extra-virgin olive oil more automatic in your prepping and cooking, keep a pourer by the stove and a dark bottle by the table. Buy your extra-virgin olive oil fresh, keep it in a dark glass bottle, check harvest/best-by dates, and store it in a cool place and use within 2–3 months of opening.

It's important to note that extra-virgin olive oil is calorie dense. Start with 1–2 tablespoons daily as a swap, not an add-on, especially when replacing butter or creamy sauces. If you have gallbladder issues or require fat restriction in your diet, reduce amounts to a tolerable level.

44

GO FOR GARLIC

To nudge liver-friendly metabolism, work garlic and its natural benefits into your routine. Garlic's organosulfur compounds (like allicin and S-allyl cysteine) boost your body's antioxidant defenses, calm low-grade inflammation, and support healthier triglycerides, LDL, and insulin sensitivity, which are key for lowering liver fat. Its gentle antimicrobial and prebiotic effects can also help you maintain a healthier gut, which leads back to a calmer, less stressed liver.

Crush, chop, or grate one to two cloves of garlic a day and use it 3 to 5 days a week. Be sure to wait 10 minutes after you crush the garlic before you heat it to maximize its production of allicin (a natural compound that supports health). Use garlic to replace salty sauces and heavy creams to give your food flavor without the metabolic load.

Try swirling raw minced garlic into olive oil and lemon for a quick vinaigrette, and then toss warm vegetables, beans, or whole grains with that dressing. Stir garlic into tomato sauces near the end of cooking, rub it on salmon before roasting, or mash roasted garlic into yogurt or hummus for a mellow spread. Roast a whole head weekly for sweet, easy flavor whenever your meals need it.

Be smart. If you have acid reflux or IBS, start with small portions and cook your garlic well. The added benefits of garlic are not present in jarred processed versions, but can be activated in powdered garlic by hydrating with a little water 10 minutes before adding it to food.

45

ADD TURMERIC DAILY TO CALM INFLAMMATION

Inflammation can silently damage your liver over time, so finding ways to combat it is key for your liver's longevity and health. Turmeric is a curcuminoid that quiets inflammation and oxidative stress, which are damaging to liver cells. It also supports bile flow and insulin sensitivity, reducing metabolic strain and fat buildup in your liver. For improved liver health, try adding more turmeric to your day by adding it to your food—and be aware that high-dose supplements can actually be harmful to your liver.

When starting to add turmeric to your routine, begin with ½ to 1 teaspoon of ground turmeric (or 1 inch fresh grated) 3 to 5 days a week. Always pair turmeric with fat and black pepper for better absorption. You can whisk it into yogurt/tahini and add a pinch of pepper, or fold it into scrambled eggs, lentils, bean chili, roasted vegetables, soups, or the cooking water for rice or quinoa. Use turmeric to replace salty sauces and heavy gravies and you'll get flavor without the metabolic baggage. You can also blend a "golden" milk (warm milk or soy milk plus turmeric, ginger, and cinnamon) or make a quick dressing of olive oil, lemon, turmeric, and garlic. Make a ready-to-use blend (2 tablespoons of turmeric and 1 tablespoon of black pepper) and keep it by the stove so adding it to your dishes becomes automatic.

If you're prone to reflux, start small and cook your turmeric well. Wipe up spills and splatters quickly, as turmeric can stain permanently.

46

EAT CRUCIFEROUS VEGETABLES

Power your liver with cruciferous vegetables like broccoli, cauliflower, Brussels sprouts, kale, cabbage, bok choy, collards, napa cabbage, arugula, watercress, radishes, turnips, and mustard greens. Recognize these brassica vegetables as natural detox partners: Their glucosinolates convert, after chopping or chewing, into sulforaphane and other compounds that help your liver neutralize and escort toxins out.

The secret to unleashing all the health benefits of these vegetables is to chop them and then wait a bit before consuming them. If you're already planning on enjoying these fiber-rich foods, you might as well get as much benefit from them as you can by simply waiting to enjoy them! Simply chop or crush your cruciferous vegetables and let them sit for 10–15 minutes to allow myrosinase to form into sulforaphane. Then lightly steam your vegetables for 3–5 minutes and try to not overboil or overcook them. You can also add a pinch of mustard powder or a handful of raw arugula to cooked broccoli to reactivate myrosinase.

Aim for 1–2 cups of cruciferous vegetables most days, rotating your colors and types. Roast Brussels sprouts, stir-fry bok choy with garlic and ginger, blend kale into smoothies, "rice" your cauliflower florets and use as a rice substitute, or build a crunchy cabbage-carrot slaw with lemon and olive oil. Stock frozen broccoli, prewashed greens, and preshredded slaw so it's easy to make your liver's favorite choice daily.

Fill your plate with cruciferous vegetables to feed your microbiome with fiber, improve insulin sensitivity, and tame your appetite—all key steps for reducing liver fat. As a bonus, you'll also bank vitamins C, K, and folate, plus antioxidant power to calm inflammation.

47

SNACK ON SEEDS

Upgrade your liver by making seeds like flax, chia, pumpkin, sunflower, sesame, and hemp some of your go-to snacks. These tiny powerhouses deliver fiber, plant protein, vitamin E, magnesium, zinc, and ALA omega-3s. In your body, they tame blood sugar spikes, improve insulin sensitivity, and lower liver fat buildup. In addition, flax and sesame seeds contain vitamin E and lignans that fight oxidative stress and support your liver's detox enzymes and healthy hormone metabolism.

Seeds also help you curb cravings with fiber-rich volume so you can naturally eat fewer ultra-processed snacks. Here are some easy ways to work more seeds into your day:

- Grind flax for ALA and lignan absorption and sprinkle 1–2 tablespoons onto yogurt, oats, or salads.
- Soak chia in water or milk for 10 minutes to form a quick pudding and then add cinnamon and berries.
- Toss pumpkin and sunflower seeds over soups or roasted vegetables for crunch.
- Whisk tahini with lemon and garlic for a quick 60-second liver-loving sauce.
- Blend hemp seeds into smoothies for creaminess without dairy.

Aim for 2–4 tablespoons of seeds daily, split across all your snacks. Keep seeds in the refrigerator or freezer to protect their oils from going rancid. Choose unsalted, unsweetened options and skip candy-coated mixes. Increase your seed intake gradually and drink water to keep digestion and your gut moving steadily. If you have a sesame or seed allergy, pick alternatives safely.

48

CHOOSE LENTILS

Lentils are a liver-loving staple. Load up on their soluble fiber and resistant starch to feed your gut microbes, generate short-chain fatty acids (like butyrate), and calm liver inflammation. Lentils have a low glycemic index that steadies blood sugar and improves insulin sensitivity, which leads to improvements in liver fat.

When you eat lentils, you get not only plant protein (approximately 15 grams per cooked cup) but also folate, magnesium, potassium, and polyphenols that support detox pathways and metabolic health. Try to replace the red or processed meat you eat with lentils to lower your saturated fat and LDL. Start with $\frac{1}{2}$–1 cup of cooked lentils daily, and drink additional water to let the fiber work smoothly in your body. You can also batch-cook and freeze portions for effortless lunches.

There are several varieties of lentils, and each has a different cooking time. You must rinse all your lentils and then cook red lentils for 12–15 minutes, cook green/brown lentils for 20–25 minutes, and cook black (beluga) lentils for 25–30 minutes. You can also try canned lentils if you are short on time; just remember to rinse them well to reduce sodium.

Here are some ideas for ways to enjoy lentils:

- Pair lentils with vitamin C foods (lemon, peppers, tomatoes) to boost nonheme iron absorption.
- Combine them with whole grains (rice, quinoa, barley) to round out your amino acids.
- Season boldly with turmeric, cumin, garlic, onion, or tomato paste to make an instant dal, soup, or chili.
- Make lentil tacos, salads, or warm bowls with olive oil and greens and let your liver win!

49

USE FRESH HERBS

Treat fresh herbs as your liver's daily upgrade. Harness their polyphenols (like rosmarinic and carnosic acids) and chlorophyll to bolster antioxidant defenses, calm inflammation, and nudge detox enzymes, all while adding flavor that helps you cut excess salt and sugar, both of which are linked to liver fat. Pile on parsley, cilantro, basil, mint, dill, chives, oregano, thyme, rosemary, and sage to make vegetables, fish, and legumes craveable.

Shop and store smart. Buy fragrant bunches of your favorite herbs, trim the stems, and stand them in a glass of water in the refrigerator (covered loosely) or wrap them in a damp towel. Wash, dry, and chop your herbs right before using them.

Next, cook strategically. Stir in delicate herbs (basil, cilantro, parsley, dill, mint) at the end to preserve their aroma and phytonutrients. Add robust herbs (rosemary, thyme, sage, oregano) earlier to infuse stews and roasts. Create a quick chimichurri, pesto, or salsa verde with olive oil and lemon and spoon over eggs, lentils, or grilled vegetables. Freeze extra herbs in olive-oil ice cubes for instant flavor bombs.

Aim for a big handful of herbs daily and add to salads, soups, grain bowls, and tacos.

50

SHOP THE PERIMETER

Fill your shopping cart where the majority of the foods that protect your liver and metabolic health live—the perimeter of the store. Start in produce and load leafy greens, cruciferous vegetables, berries, citrus, and colorful vegetables for fiber and polyphenols that lower liver fat and oxidative stress. Next, move to seafood and pick salmon, trout, or sardines for omega-3s. Then choose skinless poultry, eggs, and tofu for lean protein. Grab plain yogurt or kefir for probiotics, being sure to choose unsweetened to avoid added sugar. Finally, finish with nuts, seeds, and fresh herbs for flavors that will help you ditch sugary sauces.

When shopping, be sure to have a plan. Shop after a meal so you don't arrive hungry and overload your cart! Keep a list in your hand and commit to an 80/20 perimeter rule. Read labels on "healthy-looking" items and skip those with added sugars, refined flours, or over 10 percent sodium per serving. Avoid deli meats, bakery desserts, and sugary drinks, the major drivers of liver dysfunction. And always avoid products labeled "diet."

Make smart exceptions in the middle aisles, such as oats, brown rice, quinoa, dried or canned beans, extra-virgin olive oil, canned tomatoes, and spices. Also, be sure to choose frozen vegetables and fruit with no added sauces or syrups for budget-friendly pantry items.

Then batch-prep when you get home: Wash your greens, chop your vegetables, and cook those whole grains. Keep fruit at eye level and nuts/seeds properly portioned to avoid overeating. Make your shopping trips organized and well planned to make liver-loving food choices the easy ones.

51

EAT A RAINBOW OF VEGETABLES

Flood your liver and gut with nutrients by eating a rainbow of vegetables every day. Fill half your plate with at least four colors: red (tomatoes, red peppers), orange/yellow (carrots, squash), green (broccoli, kale, spinach), blue/purple (eggplant, purple cabbage, beets), and white/tan (onions, garlic, mushrooms).

Harness the pigments and fibers that your liver loves. Carotenoids and vitamin C fight oxidative stress, anthocyanins and betalains calm inflammation, glucosinolates from cruciferous vegetables nudge detox enzymes, and soluble fiber feeds your microbiome to make short-chain fatty acids that improve insulin sensitivity and reduce liver fat. The potassium, folate, and magnesium found in these vegetables support blood pressure and metabolic health—all positive friends of a resilient liver.

Aim for four colors at two meals daily. Here are some ideas:

- Keep a tray of colorful rainbow vegetables (peppers, cucumbers, carrots, and grape tomatoes) at eye level in your refrigerator.
- Roast sheet pans of vegetables, adding splashes of lemon and extra-virgin olive oil to boost carotenoid absorption.
- Rotate raw and lightly cooked vegetables. Steam greens 3–5 minutes, eat peppers and cabbage crisp, and pair vegetables with a drizzle of olive oil or a handful of nuts.
- Build bowls with quinoa, lentils, mixed rainbow vegetables, and herbs.

Season your rainbow vegetables boldly so their flavor is so craveable it replaces ultra-processed sides. Stay consistent and watch your energy, cravings, and labs trend better.

52

SELECT LEAN MEATS

Choose lean meats to give your liver protein without burying it in excess fat. Pick skinless chicken or turkey, extra-lean ground beef, pork tenderloin, or plant-based options like tofu and tempeh over high-fat cuts. Trim any visible fat from your meats, remove poultry skin, and opt for grilling, baking, or broiling instead of frying, which will also help bring down your calorie consumption.

Read labels and prioritize options marked "extra-lean" or with lower saturated fat per serving. Build your plate so that your portion of lean protein is palm-sized, not the whole dish. Pair with high-fiber sides like vegetables, beans, and whole grains to blunt sugar spikes and support healthy digestion, both of which ease your liver's workload.

Limit processed meats such as bacon, sausage, deli meats, and hot dogs, which also come with excess salt, preservatives, and unhealthy fats that don't do your liver any favors. Season your lean meats with herbs, spices, citrus, garlic, and olive oil instead of heavy cream sauces or sugary glazes.

Make lean choices the default at restaurants by choosing grilled fish or chicken, and ask for the sauce on the side so you can taste if you wish but also control how much you consume. By consistently selecting lean meats, you reduce fat strain on your liver and support your long-term metabolic health.

53

TRY PLANT PROTEINS

Shift more of your protein toward plants to give your liver a break while also feeding your muscles. By regularly choosing plant proteins, you lower your intake of saturated fats, which supports healthier cholesterol profiles and a better metabolic environment where your liver can repair, regenerate, and function at its best. Try building your meals around beans, lentils, chickpeas, tofu, tempeh, and edamame instead of always defaulting to meat. Start simple by swapping the usual ground beef for lentils in tacos and adding chickpeas to salads or using black beans in burritos and bowls.

Aim for at least one meatless meal per day. Treat it like an experiment and not a punishment. Try a lentil soup, tofu stir-fries, chickpea curry, or a bean and vegetable chili. These foods come packaged with fiber, which helps control blood sugar, improves gut health, and reduces the fat and toxin load your liver has to process.

Choose minimally processed plant proteins and focus on whole beans and lentils rather than the ultra-processed meat substitutes loaded with sodium and additives. When you do use tofu or tempeh, marinate them in olive oil, garlic, herbs, and spices before baking, grilling, or pan-searing. Make weeknight dinners easy by batch-cooking a big pot of beans or lentils once a week so plant protein is always ready in your refrigerator.

54

PICK WILD SALMON

Wild salmon is an excellent go-to protein over heavily marbled red meats. It is rich in omega-3s that help calm inflammation, support healthy triglycerides, and may reduce liver fat buildup. Wild salmon also provides vitamin D and selenium, which are nutrients your liver needs for repair and antioxidant defense.

Buy fresh fillets or frozen, and keep preparation and cooking methods simple. Bake, grill, or pan sear with olive oil, lemon, garlic, and herbs instead of heavy batters, sugary glazes, or buttery creams. Aim for one to two palm-sized portions of salmon per week as a part of your regular routine.

Build liver-friendly plates by pairing the salmon with roasted vegetables, leafy greens, and whole grains like quinoa or barley instead of fries, white bread, or white rice. Keep portions reasonable so that it is enough food for you to feel satisfied, not stuffed.

When shopping, choose wild-caught options when available and affordable, and rotate with other omega-3-rich fatty fish like sardines or mackerel. By regularly picking wild salmon, you tilt your diet toward healthier fats, better blood lipids, and a metabolic environment where your liver can naturally detox, heal, and perform at a higher level.

55

ADD AVOCADOS OFTEN

The monounsaturated fats in avocado support healthier cholesterol levels and may help reduce fat buildup in the liver. By making avocado a regular part of your meals, you give your liver a steady supply of healthier fats, support better lipid profiles, and create conditions for your liver cells to function and repair more effectively.

Add avocado to your meals often to give your liver healthy fats instead of the heavy, processed ones that bog it down. Slice half an avocado onto whole-grain toast, salads, grain bowls, or eggs instead of slathering on butter, mayonnaise, or creamy dressings. Use avocado as your default creamy base, and blend into smoothies or turn it into a simple guacamole with lime, cilantro, and a pinch of salt to enjoy with cuts of fresh vegetables! Swap out sour cream and heavy dips for avocado-based spreads and sauces. You'll still get that rich, satisfying texture without flooding your liver with saturated fats.

Be mindful of your avocado portions, as a quarter to half an avocado at a time is usually enough for most people. Pair it with fiber-rich foods like vegetables, beans, and whole grains to keep blood sugar steadier and reduce the metabolic stress on your liver. Keep avocados visible on your counter to ripen, and then move them to the refrigerator so they're ready for use when you are ready to enjoy them!

56

USE SPICES INSTEAD OF SALT

Use spices instead of salt on your food to protect your liver from the damage of constantly high sodium and blood pressure. Start by cutting back on how often you reach for the salt shaker, and instead try building flavors from garlic, onion powder, paprika, cumin, turmeric, black pepper, chili flakes, oregano, basil, rosemary, and thyme. Season meats, fish, beans, and vegetables generously with herbs and spices before cooking so you don't feel like you're "missing" the salt.

Clean up your "go-to" meals and make your own spice blends for chicken, fish, and roasted vegetables instead of using salty packaged mixes. Try a squeeze of lemon or lime, fresh herbs, or vinegar to brighten flavor without adding sodium. These swaps help your blood pressure, support heart health, and reduce vascular strain that can indirectly harm your liver over time.

Check labels and pick "low-sodium" or "no-added-salt" versions of broths, canned beans, sauces, and snacks. At home, rebuild your desired flavors with your spice rack and keep a few premixed jars, such as taco seasoning, curry spice blend, or Italian herbs, so they are ready for you to use. By training your taste buds to love spices more than salt, you will create a daily eating pattern that's friendlier to your liver and your whole cardiovascular system.

57

ADD CITRUS FRUITS

Add citrus fruits to your daily routine to give your liver a steady stream of supportive nutrients and fiber. Reach for oranges, grapefruits, mandarins, lemons, and limes instead of sugary desserts or ultra-processed snacks. Eat a whole orange with breakfast, squeeze a lemon over salad or fish, or drink water infused with citrus slices throughout the day.

Prioritize whole fruit over juice. Whole citrus gives you fiber, which helps control blood sugar and supports your gut, which are both crucial for easing your liver's workload. If you do have juice, keep your intake small and use a small glass, dilute it, or pair it with a protein or healthy fat so you don't get a big sugar rush.

Use citrus to upgrade meals, and use it to finish off roasted vegetables, fish, or grain bowls with a squeeze. Add orange segments to salads or mix grapefruit with avocado for a bright liver-friendly side. The vitamin C and plant compounds in citrus help with antioxidant defense, supporting your liver as it processes toxins and unhealthy fats.

Keep citrus visible on your counter, at the front of your refrigerator, or already sliced in a container so it's easy to grab. By adding citrus fruits often, you add in more fiber, antioxidants, and hydration and crowd out sugary, processed choices that make your liver work harder.

58

SPRINKLE ON CHIA SEEDS DAILY

Sprinkle chia seeds into your food daily to quietly upgrade your liver health. Chia seeds are powerhouses that deliver fiber, plant omega-3s, and antioxidants that help tame inflammation, support healthier cholesterol, and may reduce fat buildup in your liver. For every tablespoon of chia seeds you get 2 grams of protein, 3–4 grams of mostly healthy unsaturated fats, and 4–5 grams of fiber, so it's clear to see that a tiny volume of chia seeds is helpful for blood sugar, cholesterol, and liver health!

Add a spoonful of chia seeds to yogurt, oatmeal, smoothies, or salads instead of sugary granola or syrupy toppings. Start with 1–2 tablespoons per day and stir them into overnight oats, mix then into Greek yogurt, or blend them into a smoothie so they soften and form a gentle gel. This gel-like texture slows digestion that in turn steadies blood sugar and insulin spikes, which would otherwise push your liver to store more fat. Additionally, the fiber helps you feel full to reduce further snacking. Use chia pudding as a simple dessert swap: Combine chia seeds with unsweetened milk (or plant milk), a bit of vanilla, a sprinkle of cinnamon, and a small drizzle of honey or fruit on top. You get a treat that satisfies without hammering your liver with refined sugar.

Drink plenty of water whenever you use chia seeds so the fiber can do its job properly. Did you know you can even add chia seeds to your water and enjoy them in this way as well? This is especially helpful if you think your fiber intake for the day may be lacking from your food choices. Keep a small jar of chia seeds and a scoop handy on your counter so adding chia becomes automatic. By choosing chia seeds regularly, you layer in gentle fiber, healthy fats, and antioxidant support that make daily life easier on your liver.

59

STIR IN GROUND FLAX EVERY DAY

Stir ground flax into your meals and snacks to protect your liver from the inside out. By stirring ground flax into your food, you create a steady flow of fiber, omega-3s, and lignans that support cholesterol balance, hormone metabolism, and long-term liver resilience. The combination of fiber and plant omega-3s (ALA) helps lower LDL cholesterol, supports healthier triglycerides, and may reduce fat buildup and inflammation in your liver.

Use ground (milled) flaxseed, not whole seeds, so you can absorb the nutrients. Add 1–2 tablespoons to oats, yogurt, smoothies, and soups, or even sprinkle it into sauce or onto salads instead of croutons or sugary granola. Make it a nonnegotiable habit, and keep a jar of ground flax at eye-level in your refrigerator with a spoon inside so every breakfast or snack gets a quick scoop.

Mix flax into your baking by folding it into pancake batter, muffin recipes, or homemade energy bites as a partial flour substitute. You'll boost fiber and healthy fats without changing the flavor much. Always drink water throughout the day so extra fiber can move smoothly through your gut, removing waste and toxins that your liver would otherwise have to manage. Remember to store ground flax in the refrigerator or freezer to protect its delicate fats from going rancid.

60

MAKE WALNUTS YOUR GO-TO SNACK

Making walnuts your default snack feeds your liver healthy fats instead of processed junk. Walnuts are rich in plant omega-3 fats, antioxidants, and polyphenols that help calm inflammation, support healthier cholesterol, and may reduce fat accumulation in the liver. Keep a small container of walnuts in your bag, car, or desk so they're easier to reach for than chips, cookies, candy, or a sugary granola bar. Aim for a small handful (about 8–10 halves) once a day or sprinkled onto meals.

Swap out ultra-processed snacks and desserts for walnuts paired with fruit, yogurt, or a few dark chocolate chips when you want something satisfying. Use walnuts to upgrade your meals, and add them to salads, oats, roasted vegetables, or grain bowls for crunch and staying power. This helps you feel full longer, which can reduce constant grazing on sugary foods that stress your liver and metabolic health with repeated blood sugar spikes.

Buy raw or dry-roasted, unsalted walnuts most of the time and store them in the refrigerator or freezer to protect their delicate fats. By making walnuts a go-to snack, you shift your daily pattern away from refined carbohydrates and trans fats and toward nutrient-dense, anti-inflammatory fuel that supports long-term liver health.

61

HYDRATE SMART WITH COCONUT WATER

Reach for coconut water when you want something more exciting than plain water but kinder to your liver than sugary drinks. The natural electrolytes in coconut water can help with hydration, which supports your liver's ability to move nutrients, filter waste, and keep metabolism running smoothly. Use it as a step-down from soda, juice, and energy drinks that flood your system with sugar and make your liver work overtime.

When considering what type of coconut water to buy, choose unsweetened brands and treat it like a light, hydrating beverage, not a free-for-all, as it does contain some natural sugars and has a very high potassium content that can pose risks for those with kidney impairments. Pour a glass with meals or mix half coconut water and half regular water to stretch it out and soften the flavor if desired. You could also use it after a workout instead of those neon-colored sports drinks that are loaded with added sugar and dyes. You can also build simple "mocktails" with coconut water by adding lime juice and a few crushed berries or mint leaves instead of alcohol or syrupy cocktails. This lets you keep the ritual of a drink without forcing your liver to process alcohol and huge sugar hits.

Always read labels and skip brands with lots of added sugars or flavors. By using coconut water wisely, you can make a strategic swap for high-sugar, highly addictive drinks, lighten the daily load on your liver, and support healthier blood sugar and overall metabolic balance.

62

BUILD YOUR BREAKFAST AROUND OATS

Try building your breakfasts around oats to give your liver, gut, and blood sugar a gentler start to the day. The soluble fiber in oats, especially the beta-glucan, helps lower LDL cholesterol and support healthier triglycerides, which reduces the fat burden your liver has to manage. That fiber also slows digestion, smoothing out blood sugar spikes so your liver isn't fighting glucose surges all morning.

Aim for at least half a cup (dry) of oats as your base. Preferably choose rolled or steel-cut oats and not the instant packets that are loaded with sugar and artificial flavors. Cook your oats with water or unsweetened milk, and load on liver-friendly toppings like berries, chia or flax seeds, walnuts, cinnamon, and a drizzle of nut butter instead of brown sugar and syrup.

Prep your oats ahead of time to make this healthy choice easier and faster in the morning. Make overnight oats in jars with oats, milk, chia seeds, and cinnamon, then top them with fruit in the morning. Alternatively, you can cook a big pot of steel-cut oats once and then reheat portions throughout the week with a splash of water. By doing this, you can also rotate your oat toppings, so your breakfasts never feel repetitive or boring.

By building breakfast around oats, you create a steady foundation of fiber, stable energy, and cholesterol support that makes your liver's daily workload lighter and more manageable.

63

MAKE QUINOA YOUR EVERYDAY GRAIN

Make quinoa your go-to grain to help your liver process fats, manage glucose, and recover from daily stress while still feeling fully satisfied. Swap white rice, regular pasta, or buttery potatoes for quinoa several times a week. Cook a batch at the start of the week and keep it in the refrigerator so it's ready to scoop into lunches and dinners without any extra work or planning.

Use quinoa as the base for bowls and pile on roasted vegetables, beans, lentils, a lean portion of protein such as chicken or fish, and a drizzle of olive oil and lemon. Quinoa brings complete protein, fiber, and minerals that support steady blood sugar, healthier cholesterol, and less fat pressure on your liver.

Replace the usual refined grains whenever you can, and stir quinoa into soups instead of noodles or rice, toss into salads for extra protein, or mix half rice and half quinoa as a gentle transition. Season it with herbs, garlic, cumin, or a splash of low-sodium broth so its savory and satisfying flavor will appease your cravings without the need to add heavy sauces.

Rinse quinoa before cooking to remove any bitterness, then simmer it until fluffy. Keep it visible in your pantry so you reach for it first. By making quinoa your everyday grain, you shift your plate toward the fiber, protein, and micronutrients that help lighten your liver's load.

64

PICK SWEET POTATOES FOR STEADY ENERGY

Choose sweet potatoes as your go-to carb when you want to support your liver and keep your energy stable. Swap out regular fries, white rice, or plain toast for baked or roasted sweet potatoes. Their lower glycemic impact helps prevent big blood sugar spikes, which over time can drive insulin resistance and fat buildup in the liver.

Load up on the bright orange flesh of sweet potatoes and know that their color comes from beta-carotene, an antioxidant your body converts to vitamin A to further help reduce oxidative stress in liver cells. Pair sweet potatoes with a good source of protein, such as eggs, Greek yogurt, lentils, or grilled fish, and a little healthy fat, like olive oil or avocado, to slow digestion and keep you fuller longer.

Use them in simple ways by roasting a tray of sweet potatoes with olive oil and garlic to throw into salads and bowls all week. Make a breakfast hash with onions, peppers, and eggs instead of sugary cereal. When you crave comfort food, make some sweet potato wedges in the oven instead of deep-fried takeout.

Every time you choose sweet potatoes over refined carbs, you're giving your liver a calmer, steadier workload, which certainly adds up to better liver health.

65

GRAB CARROTS FOR LIVER PROTECTION

When you want to support your liver without thinking, crunch on some carrots! Use the bright orange color of carrots as a reminder that their beta-carotene is a powerful antioxidant that your body converts to vitamin A for healthy liver cells to thrive and heal. The fiber in carrots also supports healthy digestion and more regular bowel movements, which helps your body move waste products out efficiently.

Try using carrots in different ways so that eating them stays fun, easy, and interesting.

- Keep washed, cut carrot sticks at eye level in your refrigerator so they're the first thing you see when you're hungry.
- Swap chips, cookies, or candy for a handful of raw carrots paired with hummus or a small handful of nuts.
- Grate carrots into salads.
- Shave them into ribbons and use them as a salad or noodles.
- Toss carrots into a stir-fry.
- Roast them in your oven with some olive oil and a sprinkle of herbs.

Choose carrots instead of sugary snacks between meals to avoid blood sugar spikes that push your liver to work overtime. Each time you reach for crunchy carrots rather than ultra-processed snacks, you're protecting your liver and building a pattern of smart, easy wins.

66

BRIGHTEN YOUR LIVER WITH BELL PEPPERS

Pile your plate with red, yellow, and orange bell peppers to give your liver an easy, colorful boost. Bell peppers are loaded with vitamin C and other antioxidants that help reduce oxidative stress in liver cells. That means less ongoing "rust" on your system from everyday toxins, poor sleep, stress, and processed food. The fiber in bell peppers also supports regular bowel movements so your body eliminates optimally.

The more color on your plate, the more protective plant compounds your liver gets to work with. Use bell peppers as one of your go-to vegetables by adding them into omelets, stir-fries, salads, fajitas, or grain bowls, or by just eating them raw with hummus. Here are some other ideas for getting more bell peppers into your daily diet:

- Blend bell peppers and add them to sauces as a great way to get some extra fiber into your meals.
- Replace part of your pasta with sautéed peppers.
- Add them into wraps so you use less processed meat and cheese.
- Snack on sliced peppers instead of chips. Keep washed, precut strips in a clear container at the front of your refrigerator so they're one of the first things you see to grab.

Each time you add colorful bell peppers to your day, you're feeding your liver antioxidants and fiber instead of extra sugar and empty calories, and that steady pattern of healthier choices is what protects you long term.

67

CRUNCH ON CELERY TO LIGHTEN YOUR LIVER'S LOAD

Celery has very high water content, making it very hydrating for the body, and with its natural balance of sodium and potassium, it is exactly what your liver needs to flush out toxins and process everything you eat and drink.

Choose celery as a crunchy snack when you want something light in calories, filling, and liver-friendly. Wash and cut a bunch of stalks at once and keep them in a clear container with a bit of water in the refrigerator so they are always ready to grab. Reach for celery instead of chips or crackers when you want something salty and crunchy.

Pair celery sticks with foods high in protein and healthy fats, such as hummus or Greek yogurt, cottage cheese, or a natural nut butter, to turn a light snack into something more satisfying and blood sugar–friendly. Chop celery into soups, stews, tuna or chickpea salad, and stir-fries to boost volume and fiber without adding many calories.

Each time you swap a processed salty snack for crisp celery, you're trimming excess calories, added fats, and chemicals that your liver would otherwise have to handle. Those small, consistent choices are exactly what protect your liver day after day.

68

EAT WITH THE SEASONS TO EASE YOUR LIVER

Let the calendar guide your grocery cart, and your liver will thank you. Choose fruits and vegetables that are in season where you live (for example, strawberries and asparagus in the spring, berries and tomatoes in summer, squash and apples in fall, and hearty greens and citrus in winter). Seasonal produce is usually fresher, higher in vitamins and antioxidants, and lower in price, which makes it easier to fill half your plate with plants that protect your liver.

Use your local farmers' market or the "sale" section of the produce aisle as your clue to what's in season, as what's piled high and is cheap is usually the food that is in season at that time. Build your meals around those items instead of reverting to the same out-of-season choices all year. The more color and variety you can get into your diet over the year, the more different plant compounds you give your liver to work with.

Make it exciting by committing to picking one seasonal fruit and one seasonal vegetable each week to feature at home. Roast, stir-fry, or add them to salads or other dishes that you were already planning on eating. Seasonal produce often tastes better too, which will make it easier to skip those ultra-processed snacks, sugary desserts, and heavy sauces that can overload your liver.

When you eat with the seasons, you naturally eat fresher, lighter, and more liver-friendly foods without having to overthink it.

69

CHOOSE FRESH CHEESE AND SKIP PROCESSED SLICES

Choose fresh cheese as often as you can so your liver has fewer additives and less saturated fat to deal with. Reach for options like cottage cheese, ricotta, fresh mozzarella, queso fresco, or paneer instead of processed cheese slices, cheese spreads, or neon-orange shreds. These fresher cheeses are usually less processed, with shorter ingredient lists, and fewer emulsifiers your liver has to clear.

Use fresh cheese when you need a protein boost, and add a scoop of cottage cheese or ricotta cheese to fruit, whole-grain toast, or a small baked potato instead of a sugary yogurt or heavy cream sauces. Build your snacks around fresh cheeses; for example, add whole-grain crackers or greens to fresh mozzarella and tomato, or enjoy some cucumber slices topped with cottage cheese and herbs.

Watch the portion sizes and fat content of the cheese you choose, and pair it with fiber-rich foods like vegetables, beans, or whole grains to support a healthier weight. Each time you swap ultra-processed, salty cheese products for simple, fresh cheese, you're cutting back on sodium, additives, and excess saturated fats that push your liver to work overtime.

70

POWER UP YOUR LIVER WITH MUSHROOMS

Use the umami (the savory "meaty" flavor) of mushrooms to replace the usual processed meats and heavy sauces that stress your liver and make it work overtime. Use mushrooms to bulk up your meals without adding extra calories, helping with weight management and insulin sensitivity—two huge levers for fatty liver.

Take advantage of the fiber and bioactive compounds in mushrooms, which may help with inflammation and metabolic health, both key for liver protection. Slice and sauté a big batch of mushrooms with olive oil, garlic, and a pinch of salt, and store them in the refrigerator so you can toss them onto toast, eggs, or salads, or add whopping flavor to any leftover in seconds. Add them whenever you'd normally reach for extra meat, cream, or cheese in stir-fries, pasta, omelets, tacos, grain bowls, and soups. Use button, cremini, or portobello mushrooms most often, and rotate in shiitake or oyster mushrooms when you can for extra benefits.

Each time you swap a meat or creamy sauce for a generous serving of mushrooms, you're lowering the burden of saturated fat and additives on your liver while still feeling satisfied and well-fed.

EAT ONIONS OFTEN AND BOOST YOUR LIVER

Eat onions often and take advantage of their sulfur compounds, which your body uses to support natural detoxification pathways and production of glutathione, one of your liver's key antioxidant defenders. In addition, the quercetin and other antioxidants in onions help calm chronic low-grade inflammation that can damage liver cells over time. Try using red, yellow, and white onions throughout the week so you get a mix of helpful plant compounds.

Slice your onions thin and cook them gently in olive oil rather than deep-frying them. Slow sautéing helps retain flavor and avoids the burnt inflammatory fats that can stress your liver. Use raw onion in small amounts too, and add finely chopped red onion to salads, salsa, or lentil dishes. Turn onions into a kitchen base, and consider caramelizing a big pan of onions to keep in the refrigerator; then you can throw a spoonful onto eggs, vegetables, beans, or meat whenever you cook.

Each time you build flavor with onions instead of heavy cream sauces, extra sugar, or processed meats, you lower the burden on your liver while still eating food that tastes rich and satisfying.

72

TRY FREE-RANGE EGGS

Choose free-range eggs as a go-to protein to give your liver steady, clean fuel. Each egg will have approximately 5 grams of protein. The high-quality protein helps stabilize blood sugar, translating into stable insulin levels and no postmeal blood sugar crashes. Stable insulin and blood sugar means reduced liver fat production over time. Prioritize free-range or pasture-raised eggs when you can, since they tend to have more omega-3s and antioxidants like vitamin E and lutein that help calm liver inflammation.

Start your day with two eggs instead of sugary cereal, bagels, or pastries. Use the yolk (don't throw it out!) as it is a choline-rich source, and choline is a key nutrient your liver needs to package and export fat. Getting enough choline helps protect against fatty liver disease and supports healthy bile flow for digestion. Eggs were demonized in the past for raising cholesterol, but it is now understood that eggs are needed for cholesterol metabolism; however, keep in mind: Everything in moderation.

Try to eat your eggs alongside fiber, such as vegetables or whole-grain toast, to support your gut and keep cholesterol under control. Batch-cook hard-boiled eggs so you always have a quick liver-friendly snack instead of reaching for packaged processed foods. Season them with herbs, pepper, or a light sprinkle of salt instead of heavy sauces.

73

OUTSMART YOUR CARBS TO PROTECT YOUR LIVER

Stop treating all carbs as the same and start choosing them like a liver-savvy shopper. Focus on high-fiber, low–net carb foods that digest slowly and keep your blood sugar steady.

Read nutrition labels and think in terms of "net carbs" grams, which is total carbs (grams) - fiber (grams) = net carbs. Choose foods where fiber makes up a large chunk of carbs, according to the nutritional facts. Pick whole fruits, vegetables, beans, lentils, oats, quinoa, and whole-grain bread instead of white rice, white bread, pastries, and sugary snacks that spike insulin and drive fat into your liver and around your waistline. In addition, if you're having a carb, bundle it with a protein to stop that postmeal sugar spike and help you remain feeling full.

Try substituting your carbs with healthier options. For example, a great hack is to substitute your white rice for riced cauliflower. Another great substitute is to use zucchini or shirataki noodles in places of traditional spaghetti noodles. This switch has the added bonus of an increase in your fiber.

Use resistant starch to your advantage. Instead of consuming freshly made bread, rice, potatoes, or pasta, cook, cool, refrigerate or freeze, and reheat and enjoy these foods the next day. Cooling turns some starch into resistant starch, which acts more like fiber, feeding your gut bacteria and blunting blood sugar spikes, thus easing the workload on your liver.

Build your plate so half is nonstarchy vegetables, one-quarter is protein, and only one-quarter is smart carbs like beans, lentils, or whole grains. Skip sugary drinks, including juice, completely. Each smart carb choice is one less hit of sugar your liver has to clean up.

74

SKIP THE BREAD AT RESTAURANTS

At restaurants, protect your liver before your meal even arrives by skipping the bread basket. That warm, usually white bread is actually a fast sugar hit that spikes your blood glucose and insulin and signals your body to store more fat inside and outside the liver. In addition to this, much to the restaurant's advantage, it makes you *more* hungry, which may lead you to order more food than you had planned on! Instead of mindlessly snacking, decide before you sit down that you're going to pass on the bread and focus on your main meal.

Ask the server not to bring bread, or keep your hands off it by sipping still or sparkling water. If others in your party want bread, move it out of your reach. Order a side salad, grilled vegetables, or a broth-based soup to start instead. That fiber and volume will help you fill up and blunt the blood sugar rise from the rest of your meal.

Build your main course around protein (which can include fish, chicken, steak, beans, or tofu) and vegetables first, with a small portion of smart carbs like roasted potatoes, quinoa, or brown rice if you want them. Notice how you leave the restaurant feeling lighter and not stuffed and sleepy? Another tip to keep your liver health in mind at restaurants is to eat slowly and finish 80 percent of your meal, ensuring you have leftovers for another meal. Every time you skip the bread basket, you reduce a hidden sugar surge and give your liver a quieter night.

75

SEQUENCE YOUR MEALS

Use the order of how you eat your food as a simple daily step you can take to protect your liver. When you eat, follow the pattern of vegetables first, protein and healthy fats second, and starches and sugars last. Start every meal with a big portion of nonstarchy vegetables, such as salad, cucumbers, peppers, broccoli, or green beans. This fiber slows stomach emptying and creates a barrier that blunts the blood sugar spike from the rest of your meal.

Next, eat your protein and healthy fats, such as fish, chicken, eggs, tofu, beans, Greek yogurt, avocado, nuts, or olive oil–based dishes. This further steadies your blood sugar and insulin response, which reduces the amount of fat your liver is forced to store.

Only after that should you move to starches and sweeter foods like rice, potatoes, bread, pasta, fruit, or dessert. By the time you reach this part of your meal, the fiber and protein are already working to slow digestion, so your liver faces a smaller glucose rush.

Practice this meal sequencing at home and in restaurants, and arrange your plate so that vegetables are most visible and eat them first on purpose. Follow this food order habit consistently to lower insulin spikes, reduce liver fat buildup, and support long-term metabolic and gut health.

76

SLOW DOWN, CHEW, AND STOP AT 80 PERCENT

Eat slowly and treat every meal like a chance to help your liver, not hurt it. Put your fork down between bites, take smaller mouthfuls, and chew each one thoroughly before swallowing. Each chew stimulates your gut hormones to get ready to process and digest the meal that has started down the path. By chewing well, you let your body catch up, as your gut and brain need about 20 minutes to register fullness. When you rush, you overshoot hunger and dump extra calories and sugar into your system that your liver now must store as fat.

Aim to finish your meal when you are about 80 percent full. By slowing down your eating pace, this feeling or sensation will be more obvious. On a fullness scale of 1–10, stop at around 7–8. Tell yourself, "Comfortably satisfied is my goal." This reduces calorie load, blunts sugar spikes, and gives your liver less excess energy to process into fat.

Create "slow rules," such as not eating standing up, not scrolling while you eat, and trying to take a sip of water between bites. Notice flavors and textures and treat your meal like mindful eating, not shoveling. If you want a second helping, wait 5 minutes before taking it and reassess your fullness level before you do.

Practice this 80 percent technique at one meal a day, then expand. Over weeks, you'll feel lighter after meals, have fewer sugar crashes, and quietly lower the pressure on your gut, liver, weight, and metabolic health one slow, mindful bite at a time.

77

TRY A FAST

Use fasting to give your liver time off from constant processing. Start with a simple 12–14 hour fast by finishing dinner by 7:00 p.m.–8:00 p.m. and not eating again until 7:00 a.m.–9:00 a.m. In that window, your insulin levels drop and your liver can shift from storing fuel to burning stored fat and clearing waste. If this is doable and enjoyable, consider extending your fasting window to 16–18 hours.

Keep your fasting window clean with drinking water, sparkling water, black coffee, or plain tea only. Skip late-night snacks, "just a bite" desserts, or sugary drinks in the evening. Each small snack restarts insulin and keeps your liver working on duty.

During your eating window, don't binge, but instead build balanced meals with protein, fiber, healthy fats, and smart carbs so your liver isn't overwhelmed. On busy days, even pushing breakfast by 1 hour and cutting nighttime snacking is a win. Reminder to remain hydrated!

Pay attention to how you feel after your fast. Do you have more steady energy, less bloating, fewer energy crashes? If you're pregnant, have diabetes, are underweight, or take regular medications, then talk to your doctor before making big fasting changes. Start small, stay consistent, and let fasting be a gentle, sustainable rhythm that lightens your liver workload day after day.

Chapter 4

MOVE, SWEAT, AND STRENGTHEN

Exercise is just as beneficial to your liver as it is to your heart, lungs, and muscles. During physical activity, your muscles pull sugar and fat out of the blood, thus lowering the load your liver has to handle. Over time, daily exercise will improve insulin sensitivity, reduce fatty liver, and help normalize liver enzymes. This chapter gives you a variety of physical activities that you can do to match your busy schedule and current fitness level. You don't need to take on an Olympic-level training schedule to help your liver. Every kind of movement counts, and consistency will give you the best results.

78

RECORD DAILY STEPS TAKEN

Tracking your daily steps turns movement into a measurable health habit. Enable your phone's pedometer or wear a step counter. Establish a 3-day baseline. Set a realistic target of 6,000–10,000 steps a day. If you're under 5,000 steps, try to add 1,000 steps per day each week until you reach your goal. Walk 10–15 minutes after each meal to blunt glucose spikes and ease your liver's workload.

Log your steps nightly with your blood pressure, weight, and drinks consumed, and circle your best day and track your 7-day average. Here are some tips to help you get those steps:

- Try to anchor your walks to other routines, like calls, coffee breaks, transit stops, or kids' practices.
- On busy days, take a 20-minute "rescue" walk; even a 2-minute walk in your home after dinner is beneficial!
- Choose routes with hills or stairs for gentle intensity.
- Wear supportive shoes; if your joints ache, pick softer surfaces.
- Stop and seek care for chest pain, severe shortness of breath, or dizziness.
- Recruit a walking buddy for accountability, which will help motivate both you and your buddy.

After 4 weeks, reassess your energy levels, sleep quality, and waist measurement, and then raise your target or add intervals. Make steps your nonnegotiable daily action to improve your liver health.

79

MONITOR YOUR EXERCISE MINUTES

Monitor your exercise minutes to make movement a dependable and actionable liver health lever. Turn on activity tracking on your phone or watch, or consider using one of many apps available to make sure every minute is captured to help you reach your goals.

To gauge your effort while exercising, use the talk test model: Your activity is mild to moderate if you can talk during it, whereas you are unable to speak in full sentences when you engage in a vigorous activity. If doable, a combination of both types of efforts is advised to optimize all aspects of health. To optimize success and set a baseline, aim for 150 to 300 minutes a week for moderate exercise and 75 to 150 minutes for vigorous exercise. Schedule sessions in your calendar like appointments. Create a rescue plan for busy days in which you do something quick but effective, such as a 20-minute brisk walk or bike ride. Break any long sitting periods with 2- to 5-minute movement bursts, and don't forget to log them too, as every minute counts!

To log your efforts, use a simple sheet, making columns for date, minutes, steps, strength training time, and a space where you can rank your energy on a scale from 0–9. Total your minutes once a week and circle your weekly best. After 4 weeks, compare totals of your waist measurement, sleep quality, and mood, and then raise your targets. Seek care for any chest pain, severe shortness of breath, or dizziness. Know that these daily deposits of exercise will steadily lower liver fat and improve your insulin sensitivity.

80

TRACK YOUR RESTING HEART RATE

Track your resting heart rate (RHR) to turn invisible stress into a clear liver health signal. Each morning, before getting out of bed, measure your RHR with your watch or by counting your pulse at the wrist for 30 seconds and doubling it. Do it at the same time each day, before caffeine and after a full night's sleep. Log the resulting number with your sleep hours, alcohol intake, and stress level. Establish a 7-day baseline. Most adults' RHR sits between 60 and 100 beats per minute; lower rates generally reflect better cardiovascular fitness and insulin sensitivity, both of which are protective against MASLD and signs of good liver health.

Color code trends with a highlighter to make your results stand out: green within plus 3 beats per minute (bpm) of your baseline, yellow if you are 4–9 bpm above, and red if you are greater than 10 bpm above your baseline. A persistent rise usually signals poor sleep, dehydration, illness, overtraining, or excessive alcohol. Course-correct that day with water, an earlier bedtime, lighter exercise, and higher-fiber meals. Pair your RHR with step counts and exercise minutes. As fitness improves, your baseline should drift down over the weeks, which is an indicator of progress.

81

USE A FITNESS APP

Use a fitness app to make your liver care exercises more automatic and trackable. Many of these fitness apps are free, but you should pick one you like and stick with it. Don't forget to connect your phone or watch so your steps, exercise type and minutes, heart rate, and sleep synchronize without effort.

Set two goals for yourself:

1. 6,000–10,000 steps per day
2. 150–300 moderate exercise minutes per week

Add quick fields that you'll log nightly (if they are not already part of the app), including waist measurement, weight, resting heart rate, blood pressure, sleep hours, fiber (grams), sugary drinks, and alcohol units.

Then set yourself some reminders and turn them on so the app will notify you. Set reminders for:

- A 10-minute walk after meals.
- 2–5-minute move breaks every hour.
- A 9:00 p.m. wind-down to protect your sleep.

Use the app to log your food with photos; pin a widget showing today's steps, exercise minutes, and last night's sleep. Then add some color codes to spot trends: green = on target, yellow = falling behind, red = off track. Let your new fitness app be your liver health partner!

82

WEAR A SMARTWATCH CONSISTENTLY

Wearing a smartwatch to track your activity (and more!) helps you to keep your metrics in check. Wearing a smartwatch daily will make it your liver's accountability partner. Consistent activity improves insulin sensitivity, reduces liver fat, improves cardiovascular health, and even reduces dementia risk.

Many smartwatches will let you know when you've reached your targets by telling you you've closed your rings, which is a built-in reward system. Additionally, your resting heart rate (RHR) and heart rate variability (HRV) will be measured, and over time you will be able to see your trends. Here are some other ways you can use a smartwatch to improve your liver's wellness:

- Log sleep nightly and aim for 7–9 hours. Watch for low sleep efficiency. Poor sleep drives cravings and insulin resistance that stress the liver.
- Enable sedentary alerts to break up long sitting.
- Record workouts with heart rate zones.
- Use reminders for medications, hydration, and protein-rich meals that stabilize appetite.
- Track weight and waist circumference weekly via connected scales to see progress.
- Log your alcohol and caffeine intakes to spot the triggers.
- Review weekly summaries, celebrate wins, and fix one small fitness gap next week.

Wear your smartwatch, sync it, and let the data nudge you toward a lighter, healthier liver.

83

MAINTAIN A REALISTIC DAILY STEP GOAL

Count your steps like a prescription. Aiming for a set number each day, whether that be 7,000, 8,000, or 10,000, keeps you accountable and ensures consistent movement. Every step you take helps your muscles burn glucose and fat, lowering the amount that ends up stored in your liver. Over time, this reduces fatty liver, improves liver enzymes, and protects against long-term damage.

Hitting daily step goals not only supports liver health but also boosts metabolism and cardiovascular fitness. Regular walking lowers blood pressure, improves cholesterol, and increases insulin sensitivity. These changes protect your heart and reduce the cycle of buildup that drives both liver and metabolic disease.

Make your daily step goal practical. Track your steps with a phone, pedometer, or watch. Even small increases matter; for example, adding 2,000 steps a day can improve liver fat and metabolic health. Set a goal, measure it daily, and adjust as you progress. By using step goals as a simple, measurable parameter, you build habits that strengthen your liver, energize your metabolism, and safeguard your heart.

84

TRY INTERVAL WALKING

Interval walking means alternating between fast and slow paces during your walk. This simple change in pace will make your body alternate between boosting your heart rate and burning more fat, both of which improve insulin sensitivity, making them powerful tools for protecting your liver and cardiovascular health.

Try walking at a brisk pace for 1 to 3 minutes, then slow down for 1 to 2 minutes. Repeat this cycle for 20 to 30 minutes. This pattern has been shown to help your body burn stored fat more effectively than steady walking.

During your fast intervals, you should feel slightly out of breath but still able to talk. During recovery, your breathing should ease. This variation challenges your metabolism, lowers blood sugar, and reduces fat stored in the liver. Aim for interval walking three to five times a week. Use a timer, follow a podcast, or simply count lamp posts or blocks to keep your intervals easy. Interval walking is free, flexible, and an effective tool for long-term liver health.

85

DO AIR SQUATS

Use your own body weight to protect your liver. Air squats, squats done without equipment, activate your largest muscles, including your thighs, hips, and glutes. When these muscles contract, they pull sugar and fat out of the blood, lowering the load your liver has to handle. Over time, this improves insulin sensitivity, reduces fatty liver, and helps normalize liver enzymes.

The great thing about air squats is you can do them anywhere; you don't need a gym, gear, or extra time. At a desk all day? Get up every hour. Add sets of ten to twenty squats throughout the day. You can do them after waking up, during a work break, before meals, or even while on a phone call. These short bursts of strength training add up, keeping your metabolism active even when you're busy.

Stronger muscles act like a storage tank for glucose. The more lean mass you develop, the less likely excess sugar is turned into liver fat. Squats also raise your heart rate, burn calories, and help with weight management, all critical for liver protection. Drop into a squat, stand tall, and repeat. Make it a daily ritual. By adding air squats to your day, you train your body to burn fuel efficiently, strengthen metabolism, and give your liver the break it deserves. This may even energize you and make you more effective at your work, which is an added bonus!

86

TAKE THE STAIRS ALWAYS

Turn every staircase into medicine for your liver. Stair climbing combines cardio and strength training in one simple move. Each step forces your legs and glutes to work harder, pulling sugar and fat from your blood and reducing the strain on your liver. Over time, this lowers liver fat, improves insulin sensitivity, and supports healthier liver enzymes.

Skip the elevator, take the stairs at work, or set aside 10 minutes at home to climb up and down. Just a few flights a day can boost your metabolism, raise your heart rate, and burn calories quickly, helping you maintain a healthy weight, a key factor in preventing fatty liver disease. Stair climbing not only tones muscles but also strengthens your heart and lungs, improves cardiovascular fitness, improves circulation, reduces inflammation, and lowers your risk of metabolic syndrome, a major driver of liver damage. Use every opportunity to climb stairs. Treat stairs as free exercise equipment that transforms daily routines into powerful health boosters. With each step upward, you lighten the load of your liver and build resilience for your whole body.

87

TRY JUMPING TO PROTECT YOUR LIVER

Use jumping as a quick, powerful way to fire up your metabolism and support liver health. Jumping, whether simple vertical jumps, jumping jacks, or skipping rope, activates large muscle groups, raises your heart rate, helps keep your bones strong, and forces your body to burn stored sugar and fat. This lowers the amount of fat deposited in your liver and improves insulin sensitivity.

You can jump anywhere. You don't need equipment or much space. Just a few minutes of jumping each day can create meaningful changes. Short bursts such as 30 to 60 seconds at a time fit easily in between tasks or projects and can keep your metabolism active throughout the day.

Jumping strengthens your whole system, building lower body strength, strengthening bones, and improving cardiovascular fitness. The better circulation and reduced body fat it helps initiate directly lower the risk of fatty liver disease. The intensity of jumping also triggers sweating, which signals your body to burn more fuel and, in the long run, reduce stress hormones.

Protect your liver with this simple activity. Add jumping into your daily routine, such as morning warm-ups, study breaks, or workout finishers. Every leap helps your muscles utilize fat and sugar before your liver has to handle them. Jump daily and give your liver the relief it needs to stay healthy.

88

BUILD THAT MUSCLE MASS

Prioritize resistance training at least 2 to 3 days per week to turn your muscles into powerful allies for your liver. Most people do not know that around age thirty, you start to lose muscle mass. The consequences of this loss are being less strong and having a smaller reservoir of muscle to mop up circulating blood sugar as you age. It is not a coincidence that this muscle loss correlates with the development of insulin resistance and, in turn, a stressed and overworked liver.

Muscle mass loss with age, called sarcopenia, is a multifactorial process where muscle fibers shrink (atrophy) and decrease in number, driven by reduced protein synthesis, nerve cell loss, hormonal shifts, inflammation, and inactivity. All these conditions lead to weakness, frailty, and increased fall risk. This loss starts around age thirty, with a gradual decline of 3–8 percent per decade, accelerating significantly after age sixty. Prevention is key.

Focus on big, compound moves such as squats, lunges, push-ups, and rows, as these actions recruit multiple muscle groups and burn more glucose from your bloodstream. Aim for two to four sets of eight to twelve slow, controlled reps, resting 60 to 90 seconds between sets. Anchor your strength workouts to existing habits that fit your day, whether they be after school or work, so they become nonnegotiable appointments. Also, protect your sleep, because your muscle grows during deep rest, not in the gym.

More muscle means better blood sugar control, less visceral fat, steadier energy, and a stronger buffer when life throws illness or stress at your liver. Build muscle now so your liver doesn't have to fight alone later.

MAINTAIN GRIP STRENGTH

Test your grip, don't ignore it. Squeeze a stress ball, hang from a bar, or carry two grocery bags and notice how quickly your hands fatigue. Grip strength is an important snapshot of your overall muscle health and aging risk. Strong grip usually means stronger muscles, better insulin sensitivity, and lower inflammation, all of which protect your liver and brain health.

Train your grip two to three times per week. Here are some ideas for you to try:

- Try farmer's carries: Hold a heavy dumbbell or grocery bag in each hand and walk for 20–40 seconds, rest, then repeat four to six times.
- Add dead hangs from a sturdy bar for 10–30 seconds, gradually building up each time.
- Use a hand gripper or squeeze a tennis ball while you watch TV.
- Pair your grip training with full-body strength moves such as rows, pull-ups (band-assisted if needed), deadlifts, and push-ups to build the muscle mass that keeps blood sugar and liver fat in check.

Protect your hands by resting when they ache and gently stretching your wrists and fingers after sessions. Retest grip strength every few weeks using the same task, and track your progress in a notebook or app. Maintain your grip now so you can open jars, carry groceries, and live independently with a strong, more resilient liver backing you up.

90

PRACTICE BALANCING

Protect your liver by training your balance every day. Poor balance often comes from weaker muscles and slower reflexes, and these things can lead to more falls. Every fall, fracture, or hospital stay can stress your liver with medications, inflammation, and long recovery times. Guard your liver by making yourself harder to knock over.

Start small with your balance training. Stand on one leg while you brush your teeth, holding the counter if needed. Switch legs halfway. Progress to 30–60 seconds per leg without support. Add a "tightrope walk" down a hallway and walk heel-to-toe in a straight line for ten to twenty steps, looking ahead, not at your feet.

Next, layer in dynamic moves two to three times per week, including side steps, mini-lunges, and slow sit-to-stands from a chair without using your hands. Once you feel steady, practice turning your head side to side while you balance to mimic real-life distractions.

Train barefoot or in flat shoes at home to wake up the small stabilizing muscles in your feet and ankles. Track progress by counting how long you can stand on one leg and how confident you feel climbing stairs or walking in the dark. Better balance means fewer injuries and a calmer workload for your liver.

91

WALK AFTER EVERY MEAL

Protect your liver by walking for 10–15 minutes after every meal. Short, easy walks right after eating blunt the spike in blood sugar and insulin, which helps prevent fat from being stored in your liver. Research shows that even light postmeal walking can lower blood sugar more effectively than a longer walk done later. Small studies in people with fatty liver disease also suggest that regular walking improves liver enzymes and reduces liver fat over time.

Make your postmeal walks automatic. Finish eating, stand up, and head out the door or walk indoor laps. Aim for a comfortable pace, where you can talk but not sing. After a big meal or high-carb meals, extend your walk to 20 minutes.

Use these walks as a way to stack up other healthy habits, such as catching up and calling a friend, walking and talking with your partner, listening to a podcast, or doing mindful breathing. If you can't go outside, march in place, walk hallways, or climb stairs. The key is timing; move your body while your meal is being digested.

Track your progress and notice how many meals this week ended with a walk. Over months, this simple ritual can help trim your waistline, stabilize your energy balance, improve blood sugar, and unload fat and inflammation from your liver.

92

BIKE/HIKE/SWIM/RUN FOR CARDIO HEALTH

Protect your liver by making your heart and lungs work a little harder. Regular cardio exercises like biking, hiking, swimming, and running burn stored sugar, shrink belly fat, and lower liver fat and inflammation. Studies show that 150–300 minutes per week of moderate-to-vigorous aerobic exercise can improve liver enzymes and reduce fat in people with fatty liver disease, even if significant weight loss is not achieved.

Bike on a path, hike local trails, swim easy laps, or try jog-walk intervals. Aim for at least 30 minutes, 5 days a week. If that feels like too much, start with 10-minute chunks after meals and link them together over time. Use the "talk test" to measure your exertion. You should be able to speak in short sentences while doing your activity but not be able to sing.

Then, once or twice a week, try adding in short bursts of speed where you do your chosen activity faster for 1 minute and then go for 2 minutes at an easier speed. This challenges your system and improves your fitness faster. Also, don't forget to warm up for 5 minutes and cool down for 5 minutes to protect your joints and heart.

Track your distance, steps, or overall time in a notebook or app and celebrate your small wins. Every session is a deposit into your "liver health bank" by lowering blood sugar swings, trimming fat, and building a more resilient, disease-resistant body.

93

HIKE ON WEEKENDS OR YOUR DAY OFF

Protect your liver, improve your cardiovascular health, and breathe in some fresh air by turning your weekends or days off into "hiking days." Use one longer hike each week to burn through stored sugar, lower liver fat, and calm inflammation while you recharge mentally. Research shows that regular moderate-to-vigorous activity, like brisk walking, improves insulin sensitivity, trims visceral belly fat, and can reduce fat deposits in the liver over time—and it's a great way to turn exercise into an adventurous, fun event!

Pick one day and block off a 60–120-minute hiking window as if it were an appointment. Choose routes with gentle hills at first, then progress to more challenging trails as your fitness grows. Walk at a pace where you can talk in full sentences but feel your heart rate and breathing pick up.

Prepare the night before by filling your water bottle; packing a snack of fruits, nuts, and a boiled egg; and laying out supportive shoes and weather-appropriate clothing. You can even invite a friend or family member to turn your liver-health hike into a social outing.

Use these hikes to unplug from screens, connect with family and friends, breathe deeper, and de-stress (as it is proven that chronic stress hormones push fat toward your liver and waist). Track your weekly hikes, distance, and how you feel afterward. Treat each weekend hike as your "big deposit" into long-term liver protection and overall health.

94

TRAIN IN THE ZONE 2 HEART RATE

Training in your Zone 2 heart rate zone two to three times per week will protect your liver and heart simultaneously. Use this "easy but steady" cardio zone to burn more fat for fuel, improve insulin sensitivity, and lower liver fat over time. Exercise science studies show that regular moderate-intensity aerobic work (Zone 2 fitness) can reduce fat in and around the liver even without big weight loss.

Your Zone 2 heart rate is about 60–70 percent of your maximum heart rate (estimate is 220 minus your age). You can use a smartwatch or fitness tracker to help you pinpoint this point in your workout, or you can estimate it by noticing the moment you can still talk in full sentences but can't sing. If you have heart or lung issues, be sure to follow your doctor's guidance on your exercise limits.

Choose any activity you enjoy, whether it be brisk walking, light jogging, cycling, or easy swimming. Stay in Zone 2 for 30 to 45 minutes, 3 to 5 days a week. Don't forget to warm up slowly for 5 to 10 minutes and cool down for 5 minutes afterward.

Keep most of your weekly cardio in Zone 2 and save all-out efforts for occasional short bursts or interval training. While recent scientific reviews show that high-intensity exercise is superior for cardiovascular health and fitness, adding in lower-intensity Zone 2 exercises on your rest days is a win for your heart and liver. If you are not used to regular high-intensity exercise, initiating Zone 2 exercise is immensely beneficial.

Track your time in Zone 2 and notice how your pace gradually improves at the same heart rate. Build this sustainable exercise habit to smooth blood sugar swings, trim visceral fat, and offload stress from your liver for years to come.

DANCE TO BURN FAT

Dance can be an amazing aerobic workout, so protect your liver by using dance as a go-to activity for fat-burning cardio. Turn your music on and move your whole body for at least 20 to 30 minutes and then repeat it three to five times a week. Keep a pace where you can talk in short sentences but can feel your heart rate and breathing climbing.

New to trying dance? Use simple steps, side steps, grapevines, marches, arm swings, or follow an online dance workout. If you enjoy dance, join a group class and aim for a performance! The goal is continuous movement, not perfect choreography. Studies on aerobic exercise show that regular moderate-intensity activity reduces liver fat, improves liver enzymes, and boosts insulin sensitivity in people with fatty liver disease. Emerging research on structured dance programs also reports drops in blood sugar, insulin resistance, and liver enzymes after weeks of regular dance sessions. A side bonus is that the improvements in cognition produced by dancing may help to stave off dementia.

Try making dancing a consistent part of your routine by scheduling it into your day at a certain time, such as right after work, after dinner, or as a morning energy ritual. Involve your friends or family and make it a social event so it is easier to stick with. If 30 minutes feels daunting, start with 10-minute dance "bursts" and then link them together.

Track how many dance sessions you complete each week and notice how energized you feel afterward. Let the joy of movement drive consistency, while your liver benefits from lower fat, smoother blood sugars, and improved metabolic health.

96

SPRINT IN SHORT BURSTS

Your liver benefits when you sprinkle short sprints into your week. Use 10–30-second bursts of faster effort to torch your blood sugar, boost insulin sensitivity, and help reduce liver fat. High-intensity intervals like sprints have been shown to improve liver enzymes, trim visceral fat, and enhance glucose control in people with fatty liver disease and metabolic dysfunction.

Warm up for 5 to 10 minutes with easy walking, cycling, or light jogging, then do six to ten rounds of this simple pattern: Sprint (moving hard) for 10 to 20 seconds, then recover for 40 to 100 seconds at an easy pace. Keep breathing hard but in control; you should not be able to speak in full sentences during the burst.

Start with just one to two sessions per week on nonconsecutive days and keep the rest of your cardio in gentler zones. If you're older, deconditioned, or have heart, lung, or joint issues, discuss with your healthcare provider before adding sprints to your routine, and begin with brisk walking intervals instead of running.

Track how many intervals you complete and how quickly your breathing recovers. Use these brief, powerful surges as a metabolic "upgrade" that helps your liver handle sugar and fat more efficiently.

97

PRACTICE MOUNTAIN CLIMBERS

Do three sets of 30 to 45 seconds of mountain climbers, 3 to 5 days per week to spike your heart rate and improve your liver fat metabolism. A mountain climber is a simple body weight exercise that keeps your body in plank position while you bring your knees up toward your core.

1. Start by getting down on the floor on your hands and knees. Extend your legs out behind you and balance on the balls of your feet. Plant your hands directly under your shoulders with your fingers facing forward.
2. Brace your core muscles like you're about to take a punch. Your body should be in a straight line from your feet to your head.
3. Pull one knee up and toward your midsection like you're "running"; do not let your knee touch the floor.
4. Relax your midsection slightly and push your knee back toward your other foot. Straighten your leg and put it back on the ground behind you.
5. Repeat with the other leg.
6. Continue alternating your knees, adding in speed only after your form is correct.

It's important to keep your hips level, your back flat, and your neck neutral as you perform your mountain climbers. Breathe on purpose, exhale as the knee drives forward, and inhale as you switch legs. Move fast enough to sweat, but be sure to stay in control and balanced.

Finish by walking for 5 minutes to cool down and keep that glucose moving into muscle, not your liver.

98

DO GLUTE BRIDGES

Do three sets of twelve to twenty glute bridges, 3 to 5 days a week to build insulin-sensitive muscle and help reduce liver fat.

Building and activating the glutes increases lean muscles, improves whole-body glucose uptake, and reduces insulin resistance, which is one of the main drivers of fatty liver (MASLD). Resistance training like glute bridges has been shown to reduce liver fat and improve metabolic markers even without major weight loss, likely by increasing muscle-driven glucose disposal and improving insulin sensitivity.

To perform a glute bridge: Lie on your back with your knees bent and feet flat, hip-width apart. Brace your core, tuck your pelvis slightly (avoid overarching your back), and drive through your heels to lift your hips up until your body forms a straight line from your shoulders to your knees. Squeeze your glutes hard for 1–2 seconds at the top, then lower your hips slowly for 2–3 seconds. Be sure to keep your ribs down, chin slightly tucked, and knees tracking over your toes.

Then once you've mastered the exercise, progress it. Add a resistance band above your knees, pause longer at the top, or place a dumbbell on your hips. If you cramp in your hamstrings (the backs of your thighs), bring your heels closer and focus on remembering: "Heels down, glutes up."

Finish with a 10-minute walk to amplify the postexercise glucose control, and your liver will thank you.

99

TRY RESISTANCE BANDS

Use resistance bands for 10 to 15 minutes, 3 to 5 days a week to build muscle and improve insulin sensitivity, two big levers for lowering liver fat.

Resistance training improves glucose uptake by working muscles to be better "sinks" for your blood sugar, which reduces insulin resistance and fatty liver disease. Studies and clinical guidelines consistently show that regular exercise, including resistance training, can reduce liver fat and improve liver enzymes and cardiometabolic risk factors, even if the scale doesn't change much. Bands make this resistance training easier because they're joint friendly, portable, and let you accumulate high-quality weekly training volume.

To use resistance bands, loop a mini-band above your knees (or around your ankles) and keep constant tension. Don't let the band go slack. Then start with two to three rounds of twelve to twenty banded squats, twelve to twenty glute bridges, ten to fifteen lateral "monster" steps each way, and twelve to fifteen standing rows (with a long band, anchored safely). Move slowly as you release the exercise on the way down (2–3 seconds), then drive up with control. Keep your core braced as you perform the exercises, and keep your knees tracking outward so your glutes do most of the work.

End with a 5–10-minute walk to keep that glucose moving into your muscle and not the liver.

100

ADD DEADLIFTS SAFELY

Deadlift two to three sets of six to ten reps, 2 days per week to build your large insulin-sensitive muscles and support lower liver fat.

Deadlifts train the big muscle groups (glutes, hamstrings, back), which increases lean mass and improves insulin sensitivity. Better insulin sensitivity means less excess glucose and fat being shuttled into the liver, which is a key mechanism behind fatty liver disease. Resistance training like deadlifts has been shown to reduce metabolic risk markers even without major weight loss, likely because muscle becomes more effective at storing glycogen and clearing glucose from the bloodstream.

To perform a deadlift, set up by standing with your feet hip-width apart and the bar/weight close to your shins. Hinge at your hips (push your butt back), keep a neutral spine, and brace your core like you're about to cough. Grip the weight with your hands, pull back and feel the tension, then begin to stand up, pulling the weight up, and driving the floor away. Keep the bar/weight sliding up your legs, keep your shoulders back, and keep your hips and chest rising together. Finish by standing up tall, being sure not to lean back. Lower the weight by hinging first at the hips, then bending your knees once the weight passes them.

Start with a kettlebell or dumbbell, or pull foam blocks or raised plates to learn the pattern safely. Then progress slowly by adding $2\frac{1}{2}$ to 5 pounds only when your reps are crisp, and stop one to two reps before your form breaks.

101

DO KETTLEBELL SWINGS

Do six to ten rounds of fifteen to twenty kettlebell swings, resting for 45 to 50 seconds in between each rep. Repeat 2 to 4 days per week to drive a metabolic hit that supports liver fat and improves cardiovascular health.

Kettlebell swings are "power-cardio" that train large muscle groups while spiking heart rate. That combination can improve insulin sensitivity and help lower triglycerides, which are closely tied to MASLD. Consistent exercise that mixes aerobic demand and resistance work is strongly linked to reductions in liver fat and better cardiometabolic markers.

A kettlebell is different from a dumbbell and can give you some unique benefits. Its offset handle and center of mass create a pendulum when you swing it, making the hinge pattern natural and loading the posterior chain (meaning activating the muscles along the back of the body: gluteal muscles, hamstrings, and lower back extensors) through explosive hip extension. It also challenges your grip and core while letting you move fast without having to "pull" the weight up. You can swing a dumbbell, but it's harder to control, less comfortable between the legs, and often turns into an arm lift instead of a hip snap.

Begin with the kettlebell a foot in front of you. Hinge, don't squat, by pushing your hips back and keeping a neutral spine. Hike the kettlebell back, high between your thighs, then snap your hips forward hard like you're jumping. Let the bell float to chest height from hip power, not shoulder lifting. Keep your arms elevated, ribs down, and finish tall. Stop if you feel it in your low back instead of your glutes/hamstrings.

102

TRY MEDICINE BALL SLAMS

Your core, your liver, and your heart all benefit from medicine ball slams. Try to do eight to twelve rounds of ten to fifteen medicine ball slams, resting 40 to 60 seconds in between and repeating 2 to 4 days a week.

The short, intense efforts done with medicine ball slams recruit big muscle groups that improve insulin sensitivity and glucose control, leading to health benefits for your liver and beyond. Slams combine whole-body resistance (core, lats, glutes, legs) with a heart-rate spike that helps you burn through glycogen and reduces the tendency for excess energy to be stored as fat in the liver. Over time, regular high-intensity interval-style sessions are associated with improvements in triglycerides, visceral fat, and cardiometabolic risk, all of which help improve liver health.

To perform a medicine ball slam, stand tall with your feet shoulder-width apart and a soft bend in your knees. Brace your core, lift the ball overhead, and then slam it straight down by crunching your abs and hinging at the hip like you're closing a car door with your butt. Catch it on the bounce if it's designed for that, reset your stance, and repeat with speed and control. Exhale hard on each slam, and keep your shoulders stacked to protect your neck and trapezius muscles.

Scale the exercise to your needs. Use a lighter ball if your form breaks, reduce overhead height if your shoulders complain, and keep the slam powered by your hips and abs, not just your arms. You could also scale the exercise up by slamming the ball against a target on the wall, always remembering to brace your core when you do so.

103

WORK ON POSTURE MUSCLES

Train your posture muscles (upper back, deep core, and glutes) 3 to 4 days per week to make your daily movement easier and boost metabolic health that supports your liver. Stronger posture muscles reduce "energy leaks" (slouching, poor mechanics) so walking, biking, and lifting feel easier, which will translate into you naturally moving more and burning more glucose and fat. More weekly movement and muscle engagement improves insulin sensitivity and lowers visceral fat, two big drivers of fatty liver risk. Keep your posture work simple, stay consistent, and increase your resistance slowly.

Start with a 10–12-minute "posture circuit." Try two sets of:

- 10–12 band pull-aparts
- 10–12 face pulls or rows
- 20–30 seconds of dead bug
- 20–30 seconds of side plank (per side)
- 10–12 glute bridges

Move slowly, exhale on the hard part of each exercise, and keep your ribs down so your core does the work. If you sit a lot, set a timer every 45–60 minutes, and when it goes off, stand up, squeeze your glutes, and do five shoulder blade squeezes. These small reps will add up to better posture!

104

STRETCH AFTER WORKOUTS FOR MAX YIELD

Stretching for 6–10 minutes right after your workout will lock in mobility gains, calm your nervous system, and support the recovery habits that keep your liver-friendly routine consistent. When you recover better, you train again sooner, you walk more comfortably, and you keep your stress hormones lower. Regular exercise improves insulin sensitivity and reduces visceral fat, which are the main drivers of fatty liver and poor cardiovascular health. Stretching also helps you maintain good movement patterns, making strength work safer and more effective over time.

Do the following simple "postworkout reset" every training day. Breathe slowly through your nose for five deep breaths, then hold each stretch for 30–45 seconds without bouncing.

- Hip flexor lunge stretch (each side)
- Hamstring stretch
- Calf stretch
- Chest doorway stretch
- Thoracic spine opener

Keep your stretches at a mild-to-moderate tension of a 6/10 intensity, where you feel it but you can still relax. If you're sweaty and warm, this is the best time to stretch, as your tissues are more pliable and you can improve your range of motion with less strain. Finish with 60 seconds of legs-up-the-wall to bring your heart rate down and blood flow back to your brain.

105

ADD YOGA WEEKLY

Add one yoga session per week to improve your flexibility, add stress resilience, and make your liver health habits easier to sustain. Yoga helps your liver by reducing chronic stress and improving sleep quality, both of which matter because high stress and poor sleep are linked with worse insulin resistance and higher cravings. Yoga also supports regular movement by keeping joints and muscles feeling good, helping you stay consistent with walking and strength training. Less stress, better sleep, and more consistent activity all benefit your liver.

When starting your yoga practice, pick a simple plan. Choose one class (either in person or on YouTube) and do it the same day each week at the same time. Focus on poses that open tight hips and improve core control. Good poses that achieve this include downward dog, low lunge, pigeon (or figure-4), cobra, child's pose, and gentle twists. Move slowly through the poses, breathing through your nose, and aim for "steady and calm," not max intensity. If you're new to yoga, keep it at a beginner level and stop any pose that causes you sharp pain. Mild discomfort is part of growth, but sharp pain should not be. Finish with 2–3 minutes of deep breathing (longer exhales) or a short savasana. If you enjoy this, consider a "hot" class next time (see the advantages of heat in the next entry) for added benefits!

106

SWEAT IN A SAUNA

Use a sauna two to four times per week, not exceeding 10 to 20 minutes each time, to support recovery, improve cardiovascular fitness, and reinforce habits that protect liver metabolism. Temperatures associated with cardiovascular benefits range between 170°F–195°F (77°C–91°C), which are common in traditional Finnish dry saunas. Infrared saunas can achieve similar benefits at lower temperatures (120°F–150°F; 49°C–65°C) due to their ability to warm the body more deeply.

Sauna heat raises your heart rate and core temperature, creating a mild "cardio-like" stress that can improve blood vessel function and overall cardiometabolic health. Regular heat exposure also triggers activations of heat shock proteins, which help cells manage stress and may improve insulin signaling. Better insulin sensitivity and lower visceral fat are two major drivers for improving fatty liver risk. Saunas won't "detox" your liver (as your liver already detoxes itself) but they can be a powerful recovery and routine tool that keeps you exercising consistently, sleeping better, and managing stress, all of which indirectly benefit liver health.

Start conservatively with 10 minutes at a comfortable heat, then build up to 15–20 minutes as you adapt. Sit, breathe slowly, and get out if you feel dizzy, nauseous, or lightheaded. Cool down with a lukewarm shower or a few minutes of easy walking, and don't forget to rehydrate with water plus electrolytes (especially if you sweat a lot). Don't use a sauna when you're sick, pregnant, have uncontrolled blood pressure, are dehydrated, or after heavy drinking, and avoid it if your clinician has told you to limit heat exposure. Placing a cold towel on your forehead may help you tolerate the heat when trying to stay in for the recommended 20 minutes.

107

HYDRATE AFTER SWEATING

Hydrate after sweating by replacing fluids plus electrolytes so you can recover faster, keep training consistent, and protect the metabolic health your liver depends on. Dehydration spikes stress hormones, worsens workout recovery, and can make you feel fatigued and crave snacks, which may push you toward ultra-processed foods and missed workouts—self-defeating behaviors when you're trying to improve your liver and cardiometabolic health. Consistent movement and smart hydration help you show up for your next round of exercise. A bonus benefit of adequate hydration is that it supports digestion and helps your body handle higher-fiber, liver-friendly meals without feeling bloated.

Right after a sauna or hard workout, drink 16–25 ounces (approximately 500–750 milliliters) of water over the next 30–60 minutes, then keep sipping until your thirst settles. If you sweated a lot (e.g., soaked shirt, salt marks, leg cramps, headache), add some electrolytes to your water. Use an electrolyte packet/tablet or mix 16 ounces (500 milliliters) of water plus a pinch of salt and a squeeze of lemon. If you want a simple "Am I good?" check, look at your urine and aim for pale yellow within a couple of hours. Weighing yourself before and after is even better; each 1 pound (0.5 kilogram) lost is roughly 16 ounces (500 milliliters) of fluid to replace.

108

TRY HOT YOGA

Hot yoga combines heat exposure with low-impact movement that improves insulin sensitivity, stress regulation, and the habits that protect liver health. Fatty liver is strongly tied to insulin resistance, visceral fat, poor sleep, and chronic stress. Hot yoga can combat all four. The heat acts like a mild cardio stressor, while the flow builds muscle endurance and flexibility, making it easier for you to keep walking, lifting, and staying active week after week. The breathwork and downregulation at the end can also improve sleep quality and curb stress-driven cravings. Consistency beats intensity in hot yoga: Finding one hot yoga session you can repeat one or twice every week is the win.

Pick a beginner-friendly class first (slower hot flow versus an intense power class). Expect the studio temperature to hover around 95°F–104°F (35°C–40°C) with moderate humidity, hot enough to elevate heart rate and get you sweating but still safe if you pace yourself. Show up hydrated, eat light (1–2 hours before), and set one rule for yourself: Move with control, not ego. If you feel dizzy or nauseated, or if your vision narrows, rest in child's pose, sit, or step out. There are no points for suffering. Focus on big liver-friendly "builders" with steady breathing, hip mobility, glute and hamstring strength, and core stability. After class, cool off gradually and replace your fluids plus electrolytes.

109

PRACTICE FOREST BATHING

Practice forest bathing (a slow, phone-free nature walk) one to three times per week for 20 to 60 minutes to lower stress, improve sleep, and support the metabolic habits that protect your liver. Forest bathing helps improve your liver health by shifting your body into a calmer nervous system state, making it easier to sleep, recover, and stay consistent with exercise and meal planning. Forest bathing is not magic detox; it is stress control, habit support, and gentle movement that compounds over time.

Pick a safe green space such as a park, trail, or ravine and walk at an easy pace. The goal isn't steps, it's "notice and reset." Start with 2 minutes of slow breathing and engage all your senses. Look for different shades of green, listen for birds or wind, feel the air temperature on your skin, and smell the trees after rain. Every 5 minutes, pause for 30 seconds and unclench your jaw and shoulders. If your thoughts race, label what you see (pine tree, path, cloud) and return to your surroundings. Want structure? Do a "3-2-1" scan and say three things you see, two things you hear, and one thing you feel.

110

PLAY A SPORT FOR FUN AND TO LEARN

Play a sport one to three times per week just for fun and skill-building to rack up cardio, strength, and consistency—a combo your liver loves. How does sports help the liver? Sports' naturally mixed intervals (quick sprints, changes of direction) and steady movement improve insulin sensitivity and help reduce visceral fat. You also build muscle in the legs, core, and upper body, which increases your "glucose storage tank" and makes any carbs you consume easier to handle. Most importantly, sports create a community and enjoyment, which boost adherence. The best liver workout is the one you repeat.

Choose a sport you'll show up for, whether it be basketball, soccer, tennis, pickleball, skating, skiing, volleyball, rock climbing . . . anything that makes you forget you're working out. Keep it low pressure and set a tiny goal each session that could include learning a new move, improving your footwork, or practicing a serve. And let fitness be the side effect. Start with a 5-minute warm-up of an easy jog, leg swings, and shoulder circles, and then play your sport in short bursts with breaks. If you're getting back into exercise, cap your first few sessions at 30–45 minutes to avoid any soreness that may make you want to quit. Then finish with a quick cooldown and a bit of hydration.

111

WEAR A WEIGHTED VEST

Strap on a weighted vest and make your daily walk do double duty for your liver and cardiovascular health. Start light with a vest about 5–10 percent of your body weight, and focus on consistency over intensity. Walk briskly for 20 to 30 minutes, three to five times per week, remembering to keep your posture tall, ribs stacked over hips, and shoulders relaxed. Breathe through your nose when you can, and aim for a pace where you can talk but not sing.

Wearing a weighted vest helps, as the added load increases muscle activation and energy demand without needing high-impact running. This can improve your insulin sensitivity, boost glucose uptake in muscles, and support healthier fat handling—all liver-friendly moves, especially if you're trying to improve your metabolic health.

Make it safe and sustainable: Warm up with 5 minutes of easy movement, and then build up your pace. If you're sore, try again with less weight before you quit this habit. Use the vest while you do chores, take the stairs, shop for groceries, and even walk the dog. These short "mini-sessions" will add up faster than you realize.

Avoid ego-loading and remind yourself that the vest should feel like a gentle challenge and not a grind. If you have joint issues, balance concerns, or heart/lung conditions, check with your doctor before starting. If you find your current vest weight "easy," consider adding 2–5 pounds or increase your pace or incline.

112

MAXIMIZE YOUR TREADMILL WITH INCLINE WALKING

Turn a basic treadmill session into a liver-friendly metabolic upgrade by walking on an incline. Set the treadmill to a 5 to 12 percent incline (start lower if you're new), keep the speed at a brisk walk where you can still speak, and go for 20 to 30 minutes, three to five times per week. You can even entertain yourself with an episode of a show, if a screen is available, to help you reach your target time. Incline walking raises your heart rate and muscle demand without the joint impact of running, which makes it easier to stick with—and consistency is the real win for liver and cardiovascular health.

Incline walking requires more glute and hamstring participation, and those are your largest muscles. Large muscle involvement increases calorie utilization and can improve insulin sensitivity, which is a big deal because insulin resistance is tightly linked to fatty liver and metabolic dysfunction. Over time, regular incline sessions can support better blood sugar control and reduce the overflow of fat storage in the liver.

Start with 5 minutes on a flat treadmill to warm up, then alternate 2–4 minutes on an incline with 1–2 minutes flat for recovery. Keep your torso tall and avoid hanging on the rails; only light fingertip support should be considered, so that your legs do the work. Finish with 3–5 minutes to cool down, then hydrate. If your calves or low back complain, drop or reduce the incline before you contemplate quitting the session.

Chapter 5

BE SMART WITH SUPPLEMENTS AND CUT TOXINS

Your liver is a filter, purifying your blood by removing harmful and unusable elements—toxins—so the rest of your body receives only what is beneficial and necessary. Supplements can help ensure your liver is receiving enough of the essential nutrients it needs. But not all supplements are helpful, and some can even be harmful if taken in excessive amounts. They also can interfere with some prescription medications. This chapter will help you understand the various ways to support your liver with supplements and will provide practical diet and lifestyle choices that will reduce the amount of toxins your liver has to filter. Lowering your toxin load will help your liver function more efficiently, allowing it to thrive and remain healthy.

113

TRACK MEDICATIONS YOU USE

When you document all your medications, you are not only staying organized and aware, but you are also helping to protect your liver. Having a centralized list of your medications makes it easier for your doctor or other healthcare professionals to see your full health profile and make sound decisions for you should you run into any liver health issues.

Build one master list that includes prescriptions, over-the-counter (OTC) pills, vitamins, herbal supplements, protein and exercise powders, and alcohol intake. For each item, log the name, dose (milligrams), timing, start/stop dates, reason for taking, prescriber, and any possible side effects. Photograph the labels as well, and keep the list in your fitness app or notes. Don't forget to update the list the moment something changes, even if it's just a small change in dosage.

Don't forget to set guardrails for yourself. Tally your total acetaminophen intake from all sources each day and stay within your clinician's advice. Many adults target under 3,000 milligrams per day. If you have liver disease, discuss lower limits, often under 2,000 milligrams per day. If you have cirrhosis or fluid retention, avoid NSAIDs (ibuprofen/naproxen) unless your clinicians state otherwise.

Make sure your list is always the most up to date it can be. Run a weekly 2-minute audit in which you delete any stopped medications, check refill dates, and note any new symptoms. Red flag and contact your clinician urgently for yellow eyes/skin, dark urine, pale stools, right upper abdominal pain, severe fatigue, confusion, or easy bruising. Bring your up-to-date list to every appointment, and make medication tracking your liver's seatbelt—always on, quietly preventing harm.

114

KEEP TRACK OF HERBAL SUPPLEMENTS

You should treat herbal supplements like drugs and track them to protect and optimize your liver. Make a single master log with the product name, brand/lot, dose per capsule, extract ratio/standardization, start/stop dates, reason, expected effect, side effects, and who recommended it. Don't forget to photograph the labels for quick reference.

When choosing supplements keep these points in mind:

- Choose products with USP, NSF, or Informed Choice certification and avoid "proprietary" blends that hide doses.
- If you are taking supplements, add only one new supplement at a time and wait 2–4 weeks before adding another so you can tell what helps or harms.
- Flag higher-risk botanicals such as green tea extract, kava, comfrey, chaparral, usnic acid, black cohosh, and multi-ingredient fat burners, and use only with clinician guidance or skip entirely. Even small doses can cause harm.
- Watch interaction magnets such as St. John's wort or berberine, as they can alter drug levels.
- Limit your alcohol intake when trying anything new.

Review your herbal supplement list weekly, remove any duplicates, check doses, and retire anything that isn't clearly useful. Keep your list updated and see your clinician to check your liver tests, as many supplements can cause liver injury; prevention and early awareness are key.

115

KNOW BEFORE YOU SUPPLEMENT YOUR LIVER HEALTH

Use supplements as support, not as substitutes for sleep, movement, and nutrition. Start by getting your nutritional basics right, and focus on taking in adequate protein, plenty of fiber, and minimal ultra-processed foods and alcohol. If you want to add a supplement, be sure to do your research on it thoroughly and choose options with the best evidence and the lowest downside, especially if your goal is fatty liver support, improved liver enzymes, and better metabolic health.

Be wary of products sold as "liver cleanses," as they are often blends of various compounds, making individual ingredients hard to track. It's also important to know that high-dose herbals can cause drug-induced liver injury. Avoid a megadose of anything, stick to reputable brands with third-party testing, disclose your use to your clinician when having labs checked, and reassess a supplement's use after 8–12 weeks or if any new symptoms develop. If you take prescriptions, have liver disease, or are pregnant, check interactions before starting anything new.

116

KNOW THE SIGNS OF VITAMIN DEFICIENCY

It's important to know the signs of vitamin deficiencies, as they can signal liver trouble and even make it worse. Be sure to scan for early clues and act immediately. Watch for:

CLUES	RELATED VITAMIN DEFICIENCY
Easy bruising, nose or gum bleeding, rising INR (international normalized ratio—measures how long it takes blood to clot)	Vitamin K
Night blindness; dry, rough skin	Vitamin A
Fatigue, shortness of breath from anemia	Vitamins B_{12}, B_6; folate
Numbness, tingling, weak grip, unsteady gait	Vitamins E, B_1, B_6, B_{12}
Bleeding gums, corkscrew hairs, slow wound healing	Vitamin C

Also note that bile flow and fat absorption are impaired with some liver diseases, so fat-soluble vitamins A, D, E, and K may run low first. If you have bile duct issues or pancreatic disease, fat malabsorption may occur, so be sure to discuss this with your doctor and look into water soluble ADEK (vitamins A, D, E, and K) formulations.

Track any symptoms you notice with dates. Review your alcohol intake and any medications that may deplete vitamins. Ask your clinician for these targeted labs:

- **CBC/MCV:** CBC (complete blood count) is a foundational test measuring red whole blood cells, platelets, and hemoglobin. MCV (mean corpuscular volume) measures the average size of a red blood cell. Its size will give clues as to the cause of anemia.
- **B_{12}/folate:** A large average red blood cell size suggests B_{12} or folate deficiency. Knowing the levels will help target the cause and treatment strategy.
- **Vitamin D**
- **PT/INR:** PT and INR (prothrombin time and international normalized ratio) measure how long it takes for your blood to clot; these measurements are often monitored if you are on blood thinners.

Rebuild your systems with food first, including leafy greens, eggs, dairy, fish, and sun exposure. Supplement only as advised and avoid high-dose A, E, or K without supervision. Seek urgent care for severe bleeding, vision changes, profound weakness, jaundice, or confusion.

117

OPTIMIZE YOUR VITAMIN D LEVEL

Vitamin D plays a quiet but powerful role in liver health. Low vitamin D levels are consistently associated with MASLD, liver inflammation, fibrosis progression, and poorer metabolic health overall. Whereas adequate vitamin D helps regulate immune function and insulin sensitivity.

The liver is essential for converting vitamin D to its active circulating form. Your body's optimization of vitamin D starts with its absorption. Vitamin D is fat-soluble, meaning it must be taken with dietary fat to be absorbed effectively; if you take it on an empty stomach or with a low-fat meal, you can decrease its absorption by up to 50 percent. Instead, you should try to pair any vitamin D supplements with healthy fats—such as avocado, eggs, or fatty fish—for maximum absorption.

Sunlight also matters for vitamin D absorption. Sensible sun exposure, especially midday in summer months, remains one of the most efficient ways to raise vitamin D levels, though geography, season, skin tone, and age all affect production. In northern regions, supplementation is often necessary year-round.

Finally, don't forget to support the cofactors: Magnesium is required to activate vitamin D, and vitamin K_2 helps direct calcium to bones instead of soft tissues. Optimizing your vitamin D intake isn't just about bones; it's a foundational move for liver resilience.

UNDERSTAND MILK THISTLE AND ITS CLAIMS

Milk thistle, also called silymarin, is a popular supplement with multiple health claims, but as of this writing there have been no large human studies that show its use improves liver health. There are, however, some lab studies that suggest milk thistle may support liver cell resilience and antioxidant defenses. Overall, milk thistle is considered a low-drama supplement, so if this is something you want to add to your routine, it may be worth a try, provided you check with your healthcare professional first. Also, remember to pair it with good habits, such as keeping your alcohol minimal, eating 25–35 grams of fiber a day, and getting 150 minutes per week of steady movement. Think of milk thistle as the backup singer of your liver health plan and not the lead vocalist.

When looking to purchase milk thistle, buy a product that's standardized and look for silymarin or silybin on the label. Take your supplement with food to improve tolerance. A common approach is to take 200–300 milligrams, one to two times daily, for 8–12 weeks. After that time frame, reassess how you feel and what your labs show. If nothing changes, don't keep taking this supplement out of habit. Rotate it out and focus on your dietary fundamentals.

Remember to put your safety first: Skip megadose blends and detox kits. Milk thistle can also interact with some prescription medications. If you take anticoagulants (blood thinners), diabetes medications, or have complex liver disease, check with your clinician before starting this supplement. If you are maintaining the optimal lifestyle for liver health, taking milk thistle is unlikely to add any benefit.

119

DISCOVER THE TRUTH ABOUT GLUTATHIONE AND NAC

Think of glutathione as your liver's master antioxidant. It helps neutralize harmful reactive oxygen species, supports detox pathways, and protects liver cells from oxidative injury. The catch, however, is that taking glutathione by mouth has mixed and limited absorption, so results can be variable. N-acetylcysteine (NAC) is an antioxidant that reliably replenishes glutathione stores in your body. It is also commonly used to treat acetaminophen toxicity by binding to the poisonous forms of acetaminophen that are formed in the liver.

In clinical settings, boosting glutathione (directly or via NAC) is most clearly helpful when oxidative stress is driving the liver injury. In everyday liver health, NAC has the strongest practical data in people with fatty liver risk (such as excess weight, insulin resistance, and high triglycerides) because that oxidative stress is part of the MASLD/MASH pathway. Trials have shown NAC can improve liver enzymes in some populations, especially when used along with lifestyle changes. Glutathione has less consistent data.

The natural way to maximize the potential benefits of glutathione and NAC is to load up on sulfur- and glutathione-supporting foods, which include garlic, onions, leeks, cruciferous vegetables (broccoli, Brussels sprouts, kale), plus protein (eggs, fish, legumes) to supply cysteine/glycine for your own glutathione production. Then add antioxidant cofactors, such as vitamin C foods (citrus, kiwi, peppers) and selenium sources (Brazil nuts 1–2 per day, seafood) to help recycle glutathione and support glutathione enzymes.

120

ADD PRE/PROBIOTICS TO FEED YOUR GOOD BUGS

Your liver is in constant conversation with your gut through the gut-liver axis. When your gut microbiome is healthy and balanced, it keeps inflammation low, gives you better digestion, and helps regulate your immune system. You also tend to have less leaky gut permeability, fewer inflammatory by-products reaching the liver, and better bile acid and glucose regulation. Studies have suggested that adding probiotics and symbiotics (combinations of prebiotics and probiotics) can improve your ALT/AST levels, inflammatory markers, and sometimes liver fat when paired with lifestyle changes.

Probiotics are live microorganisms, usually bacteria or yeasts, that provide health benefits when consumed in adequate amounts. They are like reinforcements for your gut's existing good bacteria, often referred to colloquially as your "good bugs." Prebiotics, on the other hand, are dietary fibers that feed your good gut bacteria. They are found in foods like garlic, onions, leeks, bananas, asparagus, and oats. When your gut bacteria digest prebiotics, they produce short-chain fatty acids that have anti-inflammatory effects in the liver.

Pre/probiotics are not a replacement for medical therapy, but they can be supportive in the right patient.

Start slow with your pre/probiotic intake and then ramp up to avoid any potential bloating.

121

TRY APPLE CIDER VINEGAR

Apple cider vinegar (ACV) can blunt postmeal sugar spikes, improve insulin sensitivity, and reduce appetite in some people. Since insulin resistance is a key driver of fatty liver (MASLD), anything that helps with glycemic control can take pressure off your liver over time.

Human studies on apple cider vinegar show modest improvements in postmeal glucose and sometimes small changes in weight when used consistently with meals. Direct high-quality evidence that ACV reverses fatty liver is limited, and most "liver" claims are extrapolated from metabolic effects and animal data. So, the benefits of ACV are best framed as simple and inexpensive add-on treatments for people who are working on MASLD risk factors and not as a standalone treatment.

To incorporate apple cider vinegar into your daily routine, try a dose of 1–2 teaspoons (5–10 milliliters) or up to 1 tablespoon in a large glass of water. Drink this mixture before or with your highest-carb meal. Protect your teeth and throat from the harsh effects of vinegar by always diluting it, using a straw to drink it, and rinsing your mouth after. Vinegar can worsen acid reflux and gut motility (gastroparesis), so always use it with caution. The bottom line is that using ACV can provide a small edge for metabolic control and your liver benefits when your glucose does.

122

FERMENTED FOODS ARE FIRE

Fermented foods are a "food-first probiotic," meaning they deliver the microbes plus bioactive compounds that were created during fermentation to your gut. This is important for liver health because your gut microbiome influences inflammation, bile acid signaling, gut permeability, and the number of bacterial by-products that reach the liver through the portal vein.

Population studies repeatedly link intake of fermented food (like yogurt) with better metabolic markers, lower weight gain risk, and improved insulin sensitivity, all relevant to fatty liver. In clinical research, fermented dairy (especially live-culture yogurt/kefir) has the strongest evidence for modest improvement in lipids, glycemic control, and inflammatory markers. Direct MASLD trials using fermented foods also align with this evidence, showing that a healthier microbiome can reduce the inflammatory "load" the liver sees, especially in people with MASLD/metabolic dysfunction.

Make incorporating fermented foods into your diet a daily habit for yourself. Try these suggestions:

- Enjoy one to two servings per day of live-culture yogurt/kefir (watch added sugars!).
- Add 2–4 tablespoons per day of sauerkraut or kimchi with meals (it's also great for blood sugar!).
- Pair your fermented foods with prebiotic fiber (oats, legumes, onions/garlic, cooled rice/potatoes) so your good gut bugs stick around.

Be aware that some fermented foods may have high sodium levels, and be sure to avoid unpasteurized products if severely immunocompromised.

123

DEBUNK THE HYPE AROUND PROTEIN POWDERS

Protein powders often have a lot of unproven hype surrounding them; it's important to note that their liver benefit is mostly metabolic and body-composition driven. If you're trying to reverse fatty liver and metabolic dysfunction, the big levers are fat loss, better insulin sensitivity, and preserving lean muscle. Higher-protein diets tend to improve satiety (feeling of fullness) and help people stay in a calorie deficit. Adding resistance training with a higher-protein diet helps keep (or build) muscle, which in turn improves the glucose handling that is amazing for liver health.

In people with metabolic dysfunction, higher-protein eating patterns and whey/soy interventions have shown modest improvements in liver enzymes or liver fat markers when paired with lifestyle changes. Protein powders are a clean, predictable way to hit protein targets without all the extra carbs or fats, especially at breakfast or postworkout, when natural protein sources are not available.

Aim to get 20–30 grams of protein per meal and take protein powder once per day or as needed to meet your daily target (often 1.2–1.6 grams per kilogram per day if you're actively cutting fat and training). Pick products with minimal sugar, simple ingredient lists, and third-party testing to reduce contamination risk. If you have advanced kidney disease or unexplained elevated liver enzymes, coordinate your protein goals with your clinician. There are also scenarios where someone can be consuming too much protein, which can cause harm.

124

BEWARE OF SMOOTHIES

Smoothies can look "healthy," but they're one of the fastest ways to accidentally drink a dessert's worth of sugar in one sitting. Depending on how the smoothie is made, some can lead to liquid sugar loads, push insulin spikes, and increase triglyceride levels, resulting in your liver turning carbs into fat. So smoothies can worsen fatty liver risk even when the ingredients sound virtuous (fruit, natural juice, honey, granola).

Smoothies can become a problem because calories and sugar consumed in liquid form are less filling, easier to overconsume, and linked to poorer metabolic outcomes compared with whole foods. In terms of your liver health, the solution is simple: If you control the smoothie structure, you keep the convenience without the metabolic hit.

The red flags for smoothies include fruit juice, multiple bananas (and overdoing the amount of fruit in general), dates, honey, sweetened yogurts, "acai" bowls, or granola added on top. If you're using smoothies for weight management or for MASLD, treat each smoothie like a meal with a set recipe, not like a blender free-for-all.

A liver-friendly smoothie would include the protein first (for example, 25–35 grams of Greek yogurt/kefir or whey/soy/pea protein). Fiber next, with 1–2 tablespoons of chia/flax seeds and a handful of spinach or oats. Cap the fruit at 1/2–1 cup of berries (not, for example, 2–3 bananas plus some mango). Don't add juice to your smoothies; instead, try water or unsweetened milk sources like almond or soy. Keep the added fat optional, but you can add 1 tablespoon of nut butter for added satiety.

125

LEARN THE BASICS OF BERBERINE

Berberine is a plant alkaloid that acts like a metabolic switch to influence liver fat pathways, improve insulin sensitivity, and reduce triglycerides and LDL. In terms of liver health, this matters most for those with MASLD/metabolic dysfunction, where excess glucose and insulin resistance can drive fat deposition and inflammation in the liver.

Recent trials in those with MASLD report that berberine can lower ALT/AST, improve lipids, and improve insulin resistance markers, suggesting mild (but modest!) liver-relevant effects, especially when used as an adjunct to diet, exercise, and weight loss rather than a replacement for them. Berberine targets the same drivers you are trying to fix with lifestyle changes, including postmeal glucose control, triglycerides, and visceral fat. In studies, common dosing was 500–1,000 milligrams per day, often split and eaten with meals.

As a few cautions, you should be aware that GI upset (constipation, diarrhea, cramping) is the main side effect of berberine, and know that it is not part of the approved guidelines for liver health management. Berberine can also interact with many medications and can add to glucose-lowering, so you should check first with your healthcare provider before taking it. Always remember that supplementation is not a replacement for lifestyle changes.

126

GET SOME VITAMIN D-RICH FOODS IN YOUR LIFE

Maintaining healthy vitamin D levels is essential to optimizing liver health and is linked to a lower risk of metabolic syndrome, obesity, and cardiovascular disease. Its actions help regulate overall metabolic processes, including glucose and lipid metabolism. Vitamin D also helps suppress hepatic lipid (fat) accumulation and inflammation by activating the vitamin D receptor (VDR) in liver cells. It also exhibits antifibrotic effects, potentially slowing the progression of liver damage.

The body naturally synthesizes vitamin D from sunlight. Short, regular exposure (e.g., 5–30 minutes of sun exposure to the arms, legs, hands, and face a few times a week, ideally between 10:00 a.m. and 4:00 p.m.) can help. However, excessive sun exposure should be avoided due to skin cancer risks, and remember that sunscreen use can block vitamin D production.

Try to include foods naturally containing (or fortified with) vitamin D in your diet like:

- Fatty fish (salmon, tuna, mackerel, sardines)
- Cod liver oil
- Fortified dairy, soy, almond, and oat milks
- Fortified breakfast cereals
- Mushrooms exposed to UV light
- Egg yolks
- Beef liver

127

EXAMINE VITAMIN E

Vitamin E, a powerful antioxidant, has shown promise in improving nonalcoholic fatty liver disease (NAFLD/MASLD) by reducing liver inflammation, fat buildup, and cell damage through protecting liver cells from oxidative stress. Although the studies recommended 800 IU/day for nondiabetic adults who had evidence of liver scarring from MASLD, it didn't significantly improve fibrosis, and more research is needed before advising supplementation for long-term use.

Vitamin E isn't advised for everyone, especially those with severe liver scarring or type 2 diabetes. High-dose vitamin E supplementation was found to be associated with an increased risk of prostate cancer and has shown no benefit for preventing cardiovascular disease (CVD).

Some research suggests that dietary intake of vitamin E (from foods like nuts, seeds, and vegetable oils) may have a different, potentially protective effect than high-dose supplements, which often contain only one form (alpha-tocopherol) of the vitamin. The bottom line on vitamin E is, if you have fatty liver disease but do not have established heart disease, type 2 diabetes, liver fibrosis, prostate cancer, or a history of stroke, a daily dose of 400 IU–800 IU may provide benefit in conjunction with the lifestyle changes described in this book.

128

DRINK COFFEE

Drinking coffee, especially 3–4 cups of black coffee daily, offers significant liver protection by reducing inflammation, fat buildup (steatosis), and scarring (fibrosis). Coffee also lowers the risk of cirrhosis (even in those with alcohol-related liver disease) and liver cancer (HCC) by providing antioxidants and compounds like cafestol and kahweol that help detoxification and cell repair.

The compounds in coffee have other benefits, including protecting liver cells and detoxifying carcinogens. In addition, they also may stimulate autophagy, a process that cleans out old cell parts, improving cell function.

These reported benefits are linked to unsweetened, black coffee, as sugar and creamers can negate the positive effects. Aim for 3–4 cups daily for potential benefits, but consult your doctor, as the effects of coffee can vary. It's also wise to enjoy your last cup before 2 p.m. to avoid having the caffeine disrupt your sleep that evening.

It's a beneficial addition to managing various chronic liver conditions, though more research is needed, and it doesn't replace medical treatment.

129

CONSIDER CREATINE

Creatine supplementation shows promise for protecting against MASLD by reducing fat accumulation, but it can worsen alcoholic liver disease (ALD) and may elevate liver enzymes. While generally safe for healthy individuals, those with existing liver conditions should be cautious and consult a doctor, especially if they are consuming alcohol.

Creatine is a compound formed by three amino acids and is found in your body's muscles as well as your brain. You can get small amounts of creatine through your diet by eating seafood and red meat, but many people now take oral supplements to improve athletic performance and build muscle mass. In fact, as strength training and cardiovascular exercises grow in popularity, they come with many suggested lifestyle changes, including prioritizing protein and fiber. Supplementing with protein and creatine is now becoming a common add-on to many people's routine.

Studies, mostly in animals, suggest creatine can prevent fat buildup in the liver caused by high-fat diets and reduce inflammation and oxidative stress. Most of the research on creatine supplementation shows that it might improve age-related declines in muscle health, bone health, and performance during cognitive tasks in older adults.

Doses of creatine up to 10 grams daily for up to 5 years have been safely used (although most people stay around 5 grams daily). Side effects might include dehydration, upset stomach, and muscle cramps, and gradual increases may help reduce symptoms. Remember, as with all supplements, it is important to disclose your creatine use to your healthcare provider if any kidney issues are present.

130

COUNT YOUR CAFFEINE INTAKE AND TIMING

While coffee intake has been shown to improve liver health, caffeine is still a drug, and its dose and timing can shape your liver health and can affect your energy and sleep quality. Create a simple log to track how much caffeine you are consuming and when. Be sure to include the drink type, size, what was added to it, the amount of time since your last intake, your sleep hours, resting heart rate (RHR), and mood/energy.

Set limits and aim for under 400 milligrams per day if you're healthy. Here are some caffeine amounts in popular drinks for reference:

- Coffee (8 ounces) = 80–120 milligrams
- Espresso = 60–90 milligrams
- Tea (8 ounces) = 30–60 milligrams
- Energy drink (8–16 ounces) = 80–200+ milligrams
- Cola (12 ounces) = 30–45 milligrams
- Dark chocolate (1 ounce) = 20–30 milligrams

You need to protect sleep to protect your liver. Because caffeine's half-life is 5–7 hours, set a cutoff of no caffeine 8 hours before bedtime, or earlier if your resting heart rate is elevated. Instead of caffeine in the evening, make sure to have water, fiber-rich meals, and light exercise. In the day, pair each caffeinated drink with a glass of water, and try to minimize drinking caffeinated beverages with high levels of high-fructose corn syrup. Review your log to track weekly averages, then try to shrink doses, or move their timing earlier in the day. Make caffeine tracking your daily task for steadier glucose, better sleep, and a healthier liver.

131

CONSIDER ALCOHOL AND YOUR AGE

If you feel like alcohol hits harder in your fifties and sixties than it did in your thirties, it's not in your head. As you age, your lean mass and total water levels drop, so the same drink gets distributed in a smaller water "tank," leading to a higher blood alcohol level. At the same time, the liver shrinks and hepatic blood flow declines with age, which can further slow the liver clearing the alcohol and amplify your hangover, disrupt your sleep, and increase next-day fogginess. Older adults are more sensitive to alcohol's effects on balance, coordination, and attention, which in turn raises their fall and injury risk.

While current guidelines advise that there are no safe levels of alcohol consumption, for those who regularly drink alcohol, stopping can be difficult. Switching from "tolerance-based" drinking to "dose-based" drinking can help. To do so, you will cap your drinking at one standard drink on drinking days, and you should try to sip it slowly and enjoy it, always with food and water. Be sure to build in alcohol-free days each week and treat your sleep quality as your scoreboard of success. Recheck medications and health conditions, and know that alcohol interactions become a bigger deal with age.

132

DITCH HIGH-FRUCTOSE CORN SYRUP/SUGARY DRINKS

If you are searching for a high-impact move for fatty liver risk, make it this: Stop drinking sugar, especially sodas, sweetened coffees, energy drinks, "fruit" drinks, and anything with high-fructose corn syrup (HFCS). Liquid sugar is fast, easy to overconsume, and it pushes your liver toward de novo lipogenesis, where it turns excess carbs (particularly fructose) into triglycerides that can accumulate as liver fat.

Fructose is handled largely by the liver, and higher intake from sugar-sweetened beverages is consistently associated with greater risk of MASLD and worse cardiometabolic markers. Clinical studies show that reducing sugary beverages can lower liver fat and improve insulin resistance without any fancy supplements.

The simple rule to improve liver fat and metabolic dysfunction is to make water your default drink. Other drink options include sparkling water, black coffee, tea, or unsweetened options. If you want flavor, add lemon/lime, bitters, or a small splash of 100 percent juice, or consider some soothing broth. Read labels on foods you buy, and avoid products with corn syrup, glucose-fructose, fructose, anything ending in "-ose," and concentrate, which are common tells.

Bottom line: You cannot out-supplement a daily soda habit. Ditching sugary drinks is one of the fastest ways to help your liver de-load and detox.

133

SKIP ARTIFICIAL SWEETENERS

Zero sugar doesn't always mean zero impact. Artificial/nonsugar sweeteners (like sucralose, aspartame, saccharin, stevia blends) can keep your tastebuds locked into high-level sweetness, which can make whole foods feel less satisfying and keep ultra-processed cravings alive. The other concern is metabolic, as some literature suggests certain sweeteners can affect glucose/insulin responses and the gut microbiome. Remember, this matters because the gut-liver axis influences inflammation and liver health risk.

A recent UK Biobank report/press release found that the use of artificial sweeteners increased MASLD risk. The WHO recommends not using nonsugar sweeteners for weight control, noting that there is limited sustained benefit and potential undesirable effects. At the same time, WHO notes that replacing sugary drinks with nonsugar-sweetened beverages can help reduce calories/weight versus sugar-sweetened options, so they should be used as a bridge, not a destination.

Given the associations, use diet drinks as a short "step-down" from your usual sugary beverages, then default to water, sparkling water, or unsweetened coffee/tea. Flavor your drinks with citrus, mint, cinnamon, or berries rather than artificial sweeteners. Some go-to nonsugar sweeteners that you can use to transition to healthier habits include monk fruit, stevia, and erythritol. In addition, the recent data on allulose shows that it too could be a promising choice.

134

ELIMINATE TRANS FATS

Eliminating trans fat is a low-effort, high-return move for both your heart and liver health. Trans fat is one of the few nutrition targets that is all downside. The industrial kind (from partially hydrogenated oils) drives your LDL up, drives your HDL down, and ramps up systemic inflammation—exactly the metabolic environment that promotes insulin resistance and fat accumulation in the liver over time. When your body is chronically inflamed and triglycerides stay elevated, the liver gets stuck packaging, storing, and exporting fat nonstop—which is just fuel for fatty liver progression.

The strongest human data on trans fat is cardiovascular (it clearly worsens lipid profiles and risk), but the liver connection is straightforward; trans fat–heavy, ultra-processed diets are linked with worse metabolic health, and experimental data shows trans fats can promote liver fat buildup, oxidative stress, and inflammatory signaling. Translation: Even if you're "eating clean" in other ways, trans fats are a silent saboteur.

Scan the ingredients on all food packaging and avoid anything with "partially hydrogenated" (even if the label says 0 grams trans fats). Cut the usual suspects, like fried fast food, packaged pastries, crackers, microwave popcorn, and frosting. Replace those items with liver-friendly fats, which include olive oil, avocado, nuts, seeds, and fatty fish.

135

AVOID DEEP-FRIED FOODS

Deep-fried foods are a liver stress test. Frying at high heat creates oxidized fats and advanced glycation end products (AGEs). These compounds can ramp up inflammation and oxidative stress, which are two major drivers of fatty liver (MASLD). Fried foods are also calorie-dense and hyper-palatable, making it easy to overshoot your body's energy needs, worsen insulin resistance, and push the liver to store more fat. When the frying oils at restaurants are reused (common in restaurants), they break down even further, increasing lipid peroxides and reactive aldehydes that force the liver to do extra work to neutralize them.

Make fried foods an occasional choice and not a routine staple. If it's the crunch you're after, swap the method, not the meal you're making. Air fry, oven roast, grill, or pan sear your foods with a small amount of olive or avocado oil. Keep the breading thin (or skip it) and get the desired crispiness from spices, toasted seeds, or a squeeze of lemon plus herbs. When eating out, look for "grilled," "baked," "steamed," "broiled," or "dry-rubbed" cooking methods on the menu, or ask if the kitchen can prepare your meal in one of those ways.

136

DUMP PACKAGED MEATS

Packaged meats, such as bacon, deli slices, hot dogs, pepperoni, sausages, and jerky, can quietly undermine your liver health. These foods are often high in saturated fat and sodium that can worsen insulin resistance, water retention, and blood pressure (all common travel buddies of fatty liver). Many are also ultra-processed, meaning they come with additives like nitrites/nitrates, phosphates, flavor enhancers, and preservatives. These ingredients aren't toxic in a single serving, but frequent intake can nudge your inflammation and oxidative stress upward, exactly what you don't want if you're trying to calm liver fat, improve liver enzymes, and prevent metabolic dysfunction.

Another issue with packaged meats is that they are high in calories with low satiety (hunger satisfying) per bite. A quick sandwich can become a daily habit, displacing higher-fiber, nutrient-dense foods that support the gut microbiome. Gut health matters because a healthier microbiome helps reduce endotoxin load and inflammatory signaling that can hit the liver through the gut-liver axis.

Keep the convenience but ditch the processing. Swap deli meats for rotisserie chicken, tuna/salmon, eggs, Greek yogurt/cottage cheese, beans/lentils, or leftover roasted turkey. If you do choose packaged meat, treat it like a condiment: Use smaller portions paired with fiber (like whole grains and vegetables) and don't depend on it as your daily protein.

137

WATCH YOUR PAINKILLER USE

Painkillers are helpful to those who need them, but know that your liver keeps score. The biggest concern is acetaminophen, which is processed almost entirely by the liver. In normal doses (as per what is written on the bottle) it is safe, but frequent use, high doses, or mixing with alcohol can overwhelm liver detoxification pathways and generate a toxic metabolite that injures liver cells. The risk is even higher if you're fasting, dehydrated, have underlying liver disease, or drink alcohol regularly.

Nonsteroidal anti-inflammatory drugs (NSAIDs) like ibuprofen and naproxen don't stress the liver the same way, but they can still contribute indirectly by affecting kidney function, fluid balance, and gut integrity—factors that influence liver inflammation through the gut-liver axis.

Treat painkillers as short-term tools, not daily supplements. Use the lowest effective dose for the shortest time, and avoid stacking products that all contain acetaminophen (many cold/flu medications do). Never combine acetaminophen with alcohol, and stay well hydrated when using any analgesic. Address the root cause of the pain and simultaneous optimization (if possible) of sleep, mobility, stretching, heat/ice, magnesium, omega-3s, or topical NSAIDs when appropriate. Think of pain medications as a bridge, not a destination.

138

LIMIT YOUR SALT INTAKE

Salt isn't the enemy, but excess sodium can quietly strain your liver, especially if you have fatty liver disease, insulin resistance, or any degree of liver fibrosis. High sodium intake promotes fluid retention and can increase portal pressure (pressure within the veins of the liver), and in more advanced cases of liver disease, it can worsen swelling (edema) and ascites (abdominal fluid). Excess salt is also often a marker for ultra-processed foods that come packaged with refined carbs, unhealthy fats, and additives that drive liver inflammation.

There is also a metabolic angle to excess sodium intake; high salt diets are associated with worsened insulin resistance and higher blood pressure, both of which increase fat delivery to the liver. The liver then must manage a greater lipid load while already under inflammatory stress, an unfavorable combo.

Keep your salt use intentional, not hidden. Most sodium doesn't come from the saltshaker but is in the packaged foods, sauces, deli items, restaurant meals, and items sold as "healthy" snacks. Cook more of your foods at home and season them with acids and aromatics like lemon, vinegar, garlic, onion, herbs, spices, and chili instead of salt. These herbs and spices amplify flavor, so you need less salt.

Aim for whole foods 80 percent of the time, and always read those food labels. Any food over with 400–500 milligrams of sodium per serving should be a red flag for daily use.

139

COOK WITH CLEAN OILS

The oils you cook with matter more than most people realize, especially for liver and metabolic health. In general, using seed oils is beneficial to improving fatty liver disease, and these oils have been unjustly demonized. However, when oils are heated beyond their smoke point or reused repeatedly, they oxidize and form toxic by-products like lipid peroxides and aldehydes. These compounds increase oxidative stress and inflammation, forcing your liver to work overtime to detoxify them. Over time, this burden can worsen insulin resistance and contribute to fat accumulation in the liver.

Highly refined seed oils (such as corn, soybean, and sunflower oil) are especially vulnerable to oxidation during high-heat cooking. These seed oils are not inherently "bad" but are best used for cold or low-heat uses rather than frying or searing. In contrast, oils with more stable fat structures hold up better and generate fewer harmful by-products. Seed oils, which are rich in polyunsaturated fats (PUFAs), generally appear protective against fatty liver when compared to saturated fats. For optimal liver health, prioritize cooking in oils rich in monounsaturated fatty acids (MUFAs) and omega-3 PUFAs while limiting saturated fats. Extra-virgin olive oil (EVOO) stands out as the most evidence-supported choice, followed by canola oil, while tropical oils like coconut and palm oil should be avoided.

Match the oil to the heat. For high-heat cooking, use avocado oil, refined olive oil, or ghee, which are more heat stable. Soybean, canola, and sunflower oils are acceptable alternatives but offer fewer anti-inflammatory benefits than EVOO. For low-heat cooking or finishing, choose EVOO, which delivers polyphenols that actively reduce liver inflammation. Avoid reusing cooking oils, and don't cook past the smoke point; if it's smoking, it's breaking down.

140

AVOID PESTICIDES

Your liver is your primary detoxification organ, and chronic low-level pesticide exposure adds to its workload. Many commonly used agricultural pesticides are "lipophilic," meaning they dissolve in fat and can accumulate in body tissues, including the liver. Over time, this exposure has been linked to increased oxidative stress, mitochondrial dysfunction, insulin resistance, and high risk of fatty liver disease and metabolic dysfunction. Even doses considered to be "safe" individually can become problematic for your health through daily, cumulative exposure.

Pesticides can also disrupt the gut-liver axis through alterations in gut bacteria, increase gut permeability, and allow inflammatory endotoxins to reach the liver via the portal vein, fueling liver inflammation and impaired fat metabolism.

Reduce your pesticide exposure where it counts most. Prioritize organic options for foods known to carry higher pesticide residues (especially leafy greens, berries, apples, and grapes). When organic isn't feasible, wash your produce thoroughly, peel when appropriate, and vary your food sources to avoid repeated exposure to the same chemicals. At home, limit indoor pesticide use and opt for physical or botanical pest controls when possible.

Support your liver's natural detox system by ensuring adequate protein, fiber, and antioxidants (cruciferous vegetables, garlic, onions), and the resulting less toxic load will mean less detox strain and a calmer, healthier liver over time.

141

KEEP AWAY FROM PLASTICS IN FOOD

Plastics and your health don't mix well. Many food-contact plastics contain endocrine-disrupting chemicals, such as BPA, BPS, and phthalates. These compounds can leach into food, especially when the plastic is heated, scratched, or used with fatty or acidic foods. While human studies are lacking, animal studies have demonstrated that once inside the body, these plastics are processed by the liver, where they've been linked to increased oxidative stress, insulin resistance, and higher risk of fatty liver (MASLD). Plastics can also interfere with hormonal signaling that regulates glucose and fat metabolism. This means your liver may be pushed to store more fat while simultaneously working harder to detoxify foreign chemicals, which is a double hit to the liver. Ultra-processed foods are a major source of exposure because they are often packaged, microwaved, and stored in plastic on their journey from the factory to the table.

Treat plastic as a transport material, not a cooking tool. Avoid microwaving or pouring hot food into plastic containers. Store leftovers in glass or stainless steel, and choose fresh or frozen foods over heavily packaged options. Be cautious with plastic wrap touching food directly, especially oily foods.

Replace just one daily plastic exposure—your coffee lid/cup, water bottle, or lunch container—with a nonplastic option. Small swaps, repeated daily, meaningfully lower your liver's toxic load over time.

142

TAKE CAUTION WITH HERBAL SUPPLEMENTS

Herbal supplements are often marketed as "natural" and therefore assumed to be safe, but when it comes to liver health, this assumption can be dangerous. The liver is responsible for metabolizing nearly everything you ingest, and many herbal products place an unexpected toxic burden on this vital organ. In fact, herbal and dietary supplements are now one of the leading causes of drug-induced liver injury in North America.

Common culprits include green tea extract, garcinia cambogia, kava, turmeric (in high-dose concentrated forms), ashwagandha, skullcap, and certain bodybuilding or weight-loss blends. The risk is amplified because supplements are poorly regulated and may contain undeclared ingredients, heavy metals, or variable dosing, and some may interact with prescription medications. "Proprietary blends" are especially concerning because you don't know exactly what, or how much, you're taking.

Liver injury from supplements can range from mild enzyme elevations to severe hepatitis and, in rare cases, liver failure. Symptoms may be subtle at first but commonly include fatigue, nausea, dark urine, itching, or right upper abdominal discomfort.

Treat any supplements you take like medications. Avoid megadoses, limit the number you take at once, and be skeptical of products promising rapid detox, fat loss, or immune boosting. If you have underlying liver disease, drink alcohol regularly, or take other medications, always review any supplements you are planning on taking with a qualified healthcare professional. When it comes to your liver, "natural" does not automatically mean safe.

143

DITCH DIET FOODS

"Diet" and "low-calorie" foods are often marketed as healthy choices, but many of them undermine liver health. These products are typically ultra-processed and rely on artificial sweeteners, refined starches, emulsifiers, and chemical additives to maintain taste and texture. The liver, your body's main detox and metabolic hub, ends up doing the heavy lifting to process these synthetic ingredients.

Artificial sweeteners such as aspartame, sucralose, and saccharin have been linked in multiple studies to insulin resistance, altered gut microbiota, and increased fat storage in the liver. Rather than helping with weight loss, diet foods can worsen metabolic dysfunction, which is a key driver of nonalcoholic fatty liver disease. Many "sugar-free" snacks can also trigger cravings that can lead to overeating later in the day. Nonsugar sweeteners such as stevia and monk fruit have been shown to be liver protective and can be helpful for those wanting assistance with weight loss while changing their lifestyles.

Low-fat diet foods pose another problem. When fat is removed, manufacturers often replace it with sugar or refined carbohydrates, spiking blood sugar and increasing hepatic fat production through de novo lipogenesis. Over time, this can promote liver fat accumulation and inflammation.

Stop outsourcing your health to labels. Choose whole foods with intact fiber, natural fats, and minimal ingredients, and choose vegetables, fruit, legumes, eggs, fish, and olive oil. If it says "diet," "light," or "zero," read the ingredient list twice. For liver health, real food beats engineered substitutes every time.

144

QUIT ENERGY DRINKS

Energy drinks may feel like a quick fix for fatigue, but they can quietly strain your liver. Most energy drinks deliver a high-dose cocktail of sugar (or artificial sweeteners), caffeine, niacin (vitamin B_3), and herbal additives, all of which must be processed by the liver. Taken regularly or in large amounts, this combination can push hepatic metabolism into overdrive and affect the health of your other vital organs.

Excess sugar, especially in liquid form, is rapidly converted into fat in the liver, increasing the risk of MASLD. Even "sugar-free" energy drinks aren't harmless. Artificial sweeteners and additives may worsen insulin resistance and disrupt gut bacteria, indirectly promoting liver fat accumulation. Meanwhile, very high caffeine intake can raise stress hormones and interfere with sleep, impairing the liver's overnight repair and detoxification processes. Caffeine intake at these levels can also affect heart rhythms.

Niacin deserves special mention. While safe in normal dietary amounts, the supraphysiologic doses found in some energy drinks and preworkout formulas have been linked to elevated liver enzymes and, in rare cases, acute liver injury, especially when combined with alcohol or other supplements.

Stop chasing energy in a can. Prioritize sleep, hydration, regular meals with protein and fiber, and moderate caffeine from coffee or tea. If you need a boost, address the cause of fatigue, not the symptoms. Your liver will thank you.

145

SAY NO TO PRESERVATIVES

Preservatives help extend the shelf life of foods, but many come at a metabolic cost to your liver. These chemicals are added to ultra-processed foods to prevent spoilage, enhance color, or maintain texture, and once consumed, your liver is tasked with breaking them down and neutralizing their effects. Chronic exposure can quietly increase hepatic workload and contribute to long-term liver stress.

Common preservatives such as sodium nitrite, sodium benzoate, sulfites, and BHA/BHT have been linked to oxidative stress, inflammation, and mitochondrial dysfunction in liver cells. Nitrates and nitrites, frequently found in processed meats, are especially concerning, as they can form reactive compounds that promote liver injury and worsen insulin resistance. High-sodium preservatives also increase fluid retention and blood pressure, indirectly impairing liver and cardiovascular health.

Preservatives rarely appear alone in foods, and they often travel with refined carbohydrates, unhealthy fats, and added sugars—the famous combination associated with MASLD. Over time, this steady, toxic metabolic load can overwhelm your liver's detoxification pathways.

Instead of preservative-heavy foods, eat foods that don't have a long ingredient list. Choose fresh or frozen vegetables, fruits, unprocessed meats, legumes, and whole grains as often as you reasonably can. If you can't pronounce an ingredient or wouldn't use it in your kitchen, think twice before consuming it. For liver health, freshness is protection.

146

CLEAR OUT OLD MEDICATIONS

Keeping old or unused medications "just in case" may seem harmless but it can pose real risks to your liver. Many drugs are metabolized entirely or partially by the liver, and taking expired, duplicate, or unnecessary medications increases the chance of liver strain, toxicity, and dangerous drug interactions. Over time, this added burden can contribute to elevated liver enzymes or drug-induced liver injury.

Expired medications are especially problematic. Chemical breakdown can reduce effectiveness or, in some cases, produce by-products that are harder for the liver to process. Leftover painkillers, antibiotics, and combination cold or flu products are common culprits. Acetaminophen deserves special caution, as multiple products contain it and you could inadvertently be overconsuming it, leading to acute liver failure.

Old prescriptions may also reflect outdated dosing, conditions that no longer apply, or therapies that were meant to be short term. Mixing them with new prescriptions or supplements further increases liver risk, particularly in people who drink alcohol or have underlying liver disease.

Do a medication cleanout every 6–12 months. Safely dispose of expired or unused medications at a pharmacy take-back program. Keep a current medication list and review it regularly with your healthcare provider. Fewer, necessary medications mean less stress and more safety for your liver.

147

WATCH YOUR COFFEE ADD-INS

If your morning coffee is leaving you feeling wired, foggy, or sluggish later, it may not be the caffeine making you feel this way but what you're adding to it. Creamers, flavored syrups, sweeteners, and protein powders can frequently burden your liver, which is responsible for metabolizing fats, sugars, additives, and chemical compounds.

Many popular coffee creamers contain high-fructose corn syrup, artificial flavors, and emulsifiers. These ingredients increase liver fat accumulation, worsen insulin resistance, and can trigger inflammatory pathways. Over time, this metabolic stress may present as fatigue or energy crashes rather than obvious liver symptoms.

Artificial sweeteners, especially when consumed daily, can also disrupt the gut-liver axis. Changes in gut bacteria affect how toxins and metabolites reach the liver, potentially increasing oxidative stress.

Instead of filling your coffee with unhealthy add-ins, stick to black coffee or add a splash of real milk, unsweetened nut milk, or cinnamon. If you need sweetness, try a small amount of honey or maple syrup, used sparingly, as a little goes a long way. Pay attention to how you feel 30–60 minutes after drinking your coffee. A clear head is often a sign of your liver saying thanks.

148

AVOID BURNT OR CHARRED FOODS

That crispy, blackened edge on grilled or fried foods may taste good, but your liver pays the price for it. Burnt or heavily charred foods contain heterocyclic amines (HCAs) and polycyclic aromatic hydrocarbons (PAHs), toxic compounds formed when meat and certain other foods are cooked at very high temperatures. These chemicals must be detoxified by the liver, increasing oxidative stress and inflammatory burden.

Repeated exposure is the key problem. Diets high in charred meats have been associated with higher levels of liver inflammation and may worsen MASLD over time. For people already dealing with metabolic stress, insulin resistance, or elevated liver enzymes, this added toxic load can slow liver recovery and impair natural detox pathways.

In addition, charring your foods can negatively modify the protective nutrients, like antioxidants and amino acids, that normally support health and liver repair. What's left behind is harder for the body to process and offers less nutritional value.

The fix around this is to cook smarter by using lower temperatures, avoiding direct flames, and flipping food frequently when grilling. Marinating meats with lemon juice, vinegar, garlic, or herbs can significantly reduce toxin formation. Try to choose baking, steaming, stewing, or sautéing over high-heat grilling. Golden-brown food is fine, but blackened is a tax on your liver that you don't need to pay.

149

SAY NO TO FOOD DYES

Brightly colored foods may look fun, but artificial food dyes come with a hidden cost to your overall health. Synthetic dyes like Red 40, Yellow 5, Yellow 6, and Blue 1 are chemical compounds the liver must process and detoxify. Unlike whole foods, these dyes offer zero nutritional benefits.

Research in animal studies has shown that artificial food dyes increase oxidative stress and inflammation, both of which can strain liver detox pathways. In children and adults alike, these dyes have also been associated with headaches, hyperactivity, and brain fog, which are separate from any potential connection to the liver's handling of these chemicals. When consumed daily through drinks, candies, cereals, sauces, and even "health" foods, the cumulative exposure matters.

It is speculated that food dyes can also disrupt the gut-liver axis, as changes to the gut permeability allow more toxins to reach the liver through the portal vein, increasing inflammatory signaling and metabolic stress. For people with fatty liver disease, insulin resistance, or elevated liver enzymes, artificial dyes are an unnecessary hit to overall health.

To avoid food dyes, eat foods closer to nature and choose foods with short ingredient lists, being sure to avoid products with numbers or color names. Instead, opt for naturally colored foods using beet juice, turmeric, spirulina, or paprika. Read all your food labels; even vitamins and sports drinks can be major sources of food dyes. Your liver and body thrive on simplicity: Less color is more clarity.

150

AVOID INSTANT NOODLES

Instant noodles may be inexpensive, fast, and nostalgic, but they can promote metabolic liver dysfunction when regularly consumed. Most instant noodles are ultra-processed foods loaded with refined carbohydrates, unhealthy fats, excess sodium, and chemical additives.

The noodles themselves are often deep-fried in industrial oils before packaging. These oxidized fats promote inflammation and oxidative stress in the liver, contributing over time to insulin resistance and liver fat deposition. On top of that, the seasoning packets are sodium bombs, often exceeding half your daily recommended intake in a single serving. Excess sodium worsens fluid retention, raises blood pressure, and indirectly strains liver and cardiovascular health.

Many instant noodles contain preservatives that can disrupt gut integrity. A leaky or inflamed gut sends more toxins and inflammatory signals directly to the liver via the portal vein, increasing hepatic delivery. Over time, this gut-liver axis dysfunction can accelerate liver fat accumulation and overwhelm detox pathways.

From a nutrition standpoint, instant noodles are nearly empty calories, meaning they are low in protein, fiber, vitamins, and antioxidants, all of which your liver depends on for repair and resilience. Frequent consumption of these noodles displaces real, liver-supportive foods like vegetables, legumes, lean proteins, and whole grains.

If you are craving instant noodles but want the healthy, liver-friendly version, choose soba noodles, konjac noodles, brown rice, or lentil pasta, and build flavor with real broth, garlic, ginger, vegetables, and lean protein. Your liver will thank you.

151

TOSS OUT JUNK SNACKS

Junk snacks such as chips, candy, cookies, pastry, and packaged bars are a daily stress for your liver. These ultra-processed foods are engineered with refined sugars, white flours, unhealthy oils, and artificial additives that push the liver toward accumulating fat and inflammation.

High amounts of sugar and high-fructose corn syrup are especially harmful when consumed regularly. Unlike glucose, fructose is processed almost entirely by the liver, where excess intake is rapidly converted into fat. Over time, this drives insulin resistance and increases the risk of MASLD. Pair that with trans fats or repeatedly heated oils and you create a perfect storm of oxidative stress that damages liver cells.

Junk snacks are also low in fiber and protein, two nutrients that stabilize blood sugar and reduce liver fat deposition. Without fiber, gut bacteria shift in unhealthy ways, increasing gut permeability and delivery of inflammatory compounds to the liver.

Another hidden issue is constant grazing. Frequent snacking keeps insulin levels elevated, preventing the liver from entering repair and fat-burning mode. Your liver thrives on metabolic breaks, not nonstop processing.

Liver-smart swaps are to replace junk snacks with Greek yogurt, hummus and vegetables, fruit with nut butter, nuts, or boiled eggs. You'll reduce inflammation, feel more satisfied, stabilize blood sugar, and give your liver the breathing room it needs to heal and perform at its best.

152

SKIP KETCHUP OVERLOAD

One simple but powerful liver health hack is cutting back on ketchup. Ketchup seems harmless, but most commercial versions are packed with added sugar—often high-fructose corn syrup. That sugar load goes straight to your liver, where excess fructose is converted into fat. Over time, this can contribute to fatty liver, insulin resistance, and elevated triglycerides.

The problem with ketchup isn't the occasional squeeze on a burger; it's the hidden frequency and volume consumed, often without most even realizing it. Ketchup sneaks into fries, sandwiches, marinades, and even "healthy" meals, quietly stacking up teaspoons of sugar. Your liver has no off switch for fructose metabolism, so repeated small hits can be just as damaging as obvious sugary drinks.

The fix for ketchup overload is simple: Be intentional with it and know what you are using. Use ketchup as a garnish, not a base, and familiarize yourself with volume by measuring it instead of free-pouring. The best tip though is to swap it out entirely and instead try mustard, salsa, or a quick homemade tomato sauce using crushed tomatoes, vinegar, and spices. You'll keep the flavor without the sugar spike and develop a new healthy liver habit.

Reading labels is also essential, so be sure to look for ketchups with no added sugar or ones sweetened lightly with dates or stevia. Small changes like this reduce your liver's daily sugar burden, support better fat metabolism, and make room for real nutrient-dense foods, without sacrificing taste.

153

CUT BBQ MARINADES

While barbecue marinades taste smoky and satisfying, many store-bought versions are loaded with added sugars, refined oils, and preservatives. Much like sugary sauces, excess sugar from marinades is processed almost entirely by the liver, where it can be converted into fat and contribute to fatty liver over time.

The sneaky issue with barbecue marinades is how they are used on meat. Marinades penetrate meat, meaning the sugar doesn't drip off like sauce—it cooks in. Additionally, these marinades are often reapplied to the meat during basting, thereby doubling or tripling the sugar exposure in a single meal, all without you realizing it. This combination of sugar and high heat can also create inflammatory compounds and charring that places additional stress on liver detox pathways.

Instead of focusing on wet marinade sauces, try switching to dry rubs instead. Spices like paprika, garlic powder, cumin, black pepper, rosemary, and chili flakes add big flavor without the metabolic cost. If you do marinate your meat in a liquid solution, keep it simple with olive oil, citrus juice, vinegar, herbs, and salt.

As always, scan the nutritional labels. If sugar, corn syrup, or molasses is listed near the top of the ingredient list, skip that product. Reducing sugary marinades lightens your liver's workload, supports healthier fat metabolism, and lets you enjoy barbecue without turning a protein-rich meal into a hidden sugar bomb.

154

AVOID SUGARY YOGURT

A powerful liver health hack is avoiding sugary yogurt, and it is important to understand how misleading "healthy" labels can be. Many flavored yogurts are packed with added sugars, sometimes rivaling desserts in total sugar content. That excess sugar, especially fructose, is processed almost entirely by the liver, where it can be converted into fat and contribute to fatty liver over time. In addition, it's important to know that the "fruit" added to yogurt is often sugared and more of a jam than real fresh fruit.

The problem is perception and habit. Yogurt is often eaten daily and in large portions because it feels like a smart choice and a healthy way to start the day. After all, yogurt is packed with protein and calcium and has many favorable qualities. However, in addition to the added sugars of many yogurts, low-fat versions are even worse, since manufacturers frequently replace the fat with extra sugar to keep them palatable. This creates repeated sugar hits that stress liver metabolism.

The fix is simple and effective: Choose plain, unsweetened yogurt and customize it yourself. Add fresh berries, a sprinkle of cinnamon, vanilla extract, or a small amount of honey if you need sweetness. You'll still get probiotics, calcium, and protein—without overwhelming your liver.

Greek yogurt and skyr are especially helpful due to their higher protein content, which supports better blood sugar control and satiety. But as always, be sure to read nutritional labels carefully. If sugar is listed near the top of the ingredient list, skip it. This one swap can significantly reduce your daily sugar intake and give your liver room to recover and function optimally.

155

SAY NO TO SMOKING AND VAPING

Saying no to smoking and vaping is important to optimal liver health because what you inhale doesn't just affect your lungs, it directly impacts your liver. Every toxin from cigarettes and e-cigarettes is filtered through the liver, increasing oxidative stress and inflammation. Over time, this constant detox demand can impair liver function and worsen conditions like fatty liver disease.

Smoking reduces oxygen delivery to liver tissue and interferes with enzymes responsible for breaking down fats and toxins. Vaping, often marketed as a safer alternative, still exposes the liver to nicotine, heavy metals, and chemical flavoring agents that can disrupt normal metabolic processes. Nicotine itself promotes insulin resistance, making it easier for fat to accumulate in the liver.

The fix for this liver damage is for you to eliminate smoking and vaping entirely. If quitting feels overwhelming, start by cutting triggers—morning use, stress-related habits, or social cues. Replace them with short walks, deep breathing, or sugar-free gum to interrupt the pattern, and know that help to quit is available and guidance from your healthcare practitioner may help you reach your goal.

Supporting your quitting with proper hydration, antioxidants from fruits and vegetables, and adequate sleep helps the liver recover more quickly. Saying no to smoking and vaping isn't just about respiratory health—it's one of the most direct ways to reduce toxic load and protect your liver and body long term.

156

REFUSE PACKAGED MUFFINS

A surprisingly effective health tip for your liver and overall health is avoiding packaged muffins, even the ones labeled "organic" or "whole grain." These baked goods are often loaded with refined flour, vegetable oils, and added sugars that quickly overwhelm the liver. Once consumed, excess sugar, especially fructose, is processed by the liver and easily converted into fat, contributing to fatty liver and metabolic strain.

The danger is convenience and disguise, as packaged muffins look like a quick breakfast or snack, but many contain more sugar than a donut and are engineered to be overeaten. Because they're low in fiber and protein, they spike blood sugar, forcing the liver to work overtime to manage the fallout.

The hack is to draw a firm line: No packaged muffins. If you want something similar, make it work for your liver. Choose whole foods like eggs, Greek yogurt, nuts, or fruit paired with protein. If baking at home, use almond or oat flour, reduce sweeteners, and add fiber-rich ingredients like seeds or berries, or even consider adding in protein powder for more satiety and power.

Read nutritional labels, and if you see that sugar, syrup, or refined oils appear early on the ingredient list, it's a skip. Refusing packaged muffins reduces daily sugar load, supports steady energy, and gives your liver a break from unnecessary processing.

157

AVOID MAYONNAISE OVERLOAD

Avoiding mayonnaise overload can make a real difference for liver health, especially when most store-bought mayonnaise is built on refined seed oils and hidden sugars. Even though it may not taste sweet, these ingredients in the mayonnaise increase inflammation and place extra strain on the liver as it works to process and store excess fats.

The bigger issue is how easily mayonnaise amounts add up. It spreads fast, blends into dressings and dips, and shows up in sandwiches, wraps, and salads without much thought. What starts as a small smear can quickly become several tablespoons, quietly turning a decent meal into a heavy, nutrient-light one. Over time, that excess refined fat can slow healthy fat metabolism and worsen insulin sensitivity.

A better approach is to be deliberate and use mayonnaise when it truly adds value, not by default. Measuring instead of free-spreading helps more than you might expect. Swapping in alternatives can also change the game—mashed avocado, hummus, Greek yogurt, and mustard provide flavor and texture with far less metabolic downside.

If you do buy mayonnaise, labels matter. Short ingredient lists and oils like olive or avocado are better choices. Keeping mayonnaise in check reduces unnecessary fat load and gives your liver more room to do what it does best.

158

RESEARCH OBESITY MEDICATIONS AND MASH

Recent targeted drug therapies for obesity and type 2 diabetes management have shown not only improvements in weight and diabetes biometrics but also benefits for liver conditions, including the reversal of MASLD and associated liver fibrosis (MASH).

In patients with MASLD, semaglutides seem to help by reducing fat buildup in the liver, improving how the body is using insulin and lowering inflammation. Some clinical trials have also shown that it can reduce liver scarring. In one recent study, many patients showed improved liver tissue and a reduction in key liver damage markers.

Pharmacologic therapy for MASH is rapidly evolving, with GLP-1 agonists like semaglutide (Wegovy, Ozempic) being shown to be highly effective for resolving MASH and fibrosis, and semaglutide gaining FDA approval for MASH in August 2025. In addition, resmetirom (a thyroid hormone receptor beta agonist) was approved by the FDA for MASH with fibrosis (stages 2–3) in 2024.

Discuss with your healthcare provider to determine if you would benefit from these medications. These often easily available medications have the potential to prevent liver cirrhosis and similarly improve cardiometabolic health, weight, and liver health in those who have stage 2–3 liver fibrosis. More studies are underway to identify the effect of combining therapies in those with established cirrhosis.

Chapter 6

PROTECT YOUR LIVER WITH PROPER REST

Proper rest is an essential, but often overlooked or neglected, part of maintaining your liver health. Sleep gives your liver the time it needs to perform routine maintenance that sustains day-to-day function and repair any damage that has occurred. While you sleep, your body is still hard at work performing functions that can only be done while you are at rest. This chapter will help you find practical ways to get the rest you and your liver need and deserve. And as a bonus, you may find the hacks will help lower your stress level, increase your energy level, and leave you with a greater sense of well-being.

159

SLEEP YOUR WAY TO LIVER REPAIR

Sleep plays a bigger role in liver repair than most people realize. The liver follows a strong circadian rhythm, doing much of its detox and repair work while you're asleep. When sleep is short or irregular, those processes get disrupted, making it harder for the liver to clear toxins, regulate blood sugar, and manage fat.

Poor sleep increases cortisol and insulin resistance, both of which push more fat toward the liver. Even 1 or 2 bad nights can raise inflammation and slow liver enzyme function. Over time, chronic sleep debt quietly compounds other lifestyle stressors like sugar, alcohol, and ultra-processed foods.

The goal isn't perfection, it's consistency. Going to bed and waking up at roughly the same time each day helps synchronize liver activity. A dark, cool room supports deeper sleep stages, when cellular repair is most active. Limiting late-night eating is another underrated move; giving the liver a break from digestion allows it to focus on cleanup instead of calorie processing and even affects your food choices and energy expenditure the next day.

Simple habits add up. Reduce screen time before bed, keep caffeine earlier in the day, and get morning sunlight to anchor your sleep cycle. Prioritizing sleep isn't passive or lazy; it's one of the most effective ways to support liver recovery and long-term metabolic health.

160

TRACK HOURS OF QUALITY SLEEP

Better sleep tightens your insulin control, steadies cravings, and lightens your liver's load, so it's important to know how much sleep, and how good a sleep, you are getting. To get an idea of your sleep patterns and consistency, try tracking your nightly sleep hours and their quality. Create a 7-day log and record your bedtime, wake time, total sleep hours, and awakenings (using your phone/smartwatch). Aim to get 7–9 hours per night.

Next, add some simple quality markers: sleep efficiency (time asleep divided by total time in bed; target 85 percent), your resting heart rate (RHR) on waking, and a morning energy score (on a scale of 0–10). Then color code the results as follows:

- Green = over 7 hours, 85 percent efficiency
- Yellow = 6–6.9 hours, 75–84 percent efficiency
- Red = under 6 hours, less than 75 percent efficiency; over three awakenings

Next, based on the data you collect, try these responses:

- If your results were in red: Skip alcohol, avoid late meals, walk after meals, and hydrate.
- If your results were in yellow: Keep exercise easy to moderate and make your bedtime earlier by 30 minutes. Lock in sleep anchors, which include keeping the same wake time daily, last meal more than 3 hours before bedtime, screens off 60 minutes before lights out, and keeping your room cool and dark.

Review your data weekly and track 7- and 28-day averages. Log snoring, gasping, or daytime sleepiness, and seek a medical review for possible sleep apnea.

161

GET SCREENED FOR SLEEP APNEA

Sleep apnea, or episodes of not breathing, leads to repeated drops in blood oxygen levels. This process drives insulin resistance, fat buildup, inflammation, and fibrosis in the liver. Treat any snoring, gasping, or unrefreshing sleep as red flags. Your action plan: Screen, test, treat, and track so nighttime breathing doesn't sabotage your liver and cardiovascular health.

Screen yourself with the STOP-BANG questionnaire by counting how many of the following items affect you:

- S – snoring (do you snore loudly?)
- T – tired (do you often feel tired or sleepy during the day?)
- O – observed apneas (has anyone observed you stop breathing or choke/gasp during sleep?)
- P – pressure (do you have high blood pressure?)
- B – BMI (do you have a BMI higher than 35?)
- A – age (are you older than 50?)
- N – neck (thick) (is your shirt collar 16 inches or larger?)
- G – gender (are you male?)

If your score is 0–2, you are at low risk.

If your score is 3–4, you are at intermediate risk, and you should book some testing.

If your score is 5–9, you are at a high risk, and you should get tested as soon as possible.

Ask your clinician which sleep apnea study best fits your situation. If diagnosed, use therapy nightly such as CPAP (continuous positive airway pressure). Pair this with weight management, alcohol reduction, and postmeal walks—behaviors that lower liver fat and improve insulin sensitivity.

162

NAP SMART, NOT LONG

Short, well-timed naps can support liver health, but long or poorly timed ones often backfire. The liver runs on a daily rhythm, closely tied to sleep and wake cycles. When naps stretch too long or happen late in the day, they can disrupt nighttime sleep, which is when most liver repair and detox work happens.

Extended naps can also signal or worsen poor sleep quality at night, leading to higher insulin resistance and inflammation. That combination encourages fat buildup in the liver and makes it harder for the body to regulate blood sugar efficiently. What feels like extra rest can quietly interfere with the liver's natural recovery window.

Smarter naps are brief and intentional, and it is advised that if you are napping, you should aim for 10–30 minutes, ideally in the early afternoon. This window can restore alertness and reduce stress hormones without pushing you into deeper sleep stages that leave you groggy and disrupt your evening routine.

It is important to also pay attention to the reason you're napping. If exhaustion is constant, it may be a sign of poor nighttime sleep, late meals, or blood sugar swings—all of which affect liver function. Poor nighttime sleep can be affected by alcohol intake, caffeine, or even undiagnosed sleep apnea. Used wisely, short naps can support energy and stress balance. Used poorly, they can work against the very systems you're trying to protect.

163

PRACTICE DEEP BREATHING

Practicing deep breathing for 5 minutes a day helps lower stress, improve sleep readiness, and make liver-friendly choices easier to stick with.

Your liver benefits from deep breathing through a few mechanisms. First, stress from life can push cortisol higher, which can worsen insulin resistance, increase abdominal fat storage, and drive cravings for ultra-processed foods—all patterns that raise fatty liver risk. Deep breathing also activates your parasympathetic "rest and digest" system, which helps your heart rate settle and helps normalize appetite cues. Better stress control also improves sleep quality, and better sleep supports healthier glucose control the next day and optimizes your wellness and energy to be more active. Deep breathing is a small habit with compounding effects.

Use this simple method to practice deep breathing:

1. Keeping your shoulders relaxed, inhale through your nose for 4 seconds. Let your belly expand on the inhale (allowing your diaphragm to work).
2. Exhale slowly for 6–8 seconds.
3. Do twenty to thirty total breaths.

If your mind wanders as you are breathing, just return to your counting—it's no big deal and do not let this add any stress.

Try this at the highest leverage times, which are right when you wake up, before you eat, when you're feeling stressed, and 10 minutes before bed. Want an even faster "reset"? Do two physiological sighs: Inhale, top up with a quick second inhale, then a long exhale. Repeat this three to five times.

164

TURN OFF SCREENS, TURN ON RECOVERY

Turning off screens earlier in the evening plays a quiet but important role in recovery, including how well your liver functions. Blue light from phones, tablets, and TVs suppresses melatonin, the hormone that signals your body it's time to rest. When melatonin is delayed, sleep quality drops—and the liver loses valuable time for repair and detox work.

Late-night scrolling also keeps the brain stimulated and stress hormones elevated. That combination interferes with deep sleep, raises insulin resistance, and promotes inflammation, all of which increase the liver's workload. Even if total sleep time looks adequate on paper, screen-heavy evenings often lead to lighter, less restorative sleep.

The shift doesn't have to be extreme, and even powering down screens 60–90 minutes before bed can noticeably improve sleep depth. Use warmer lighting, read, stretch, or wind down with calm music instead. If screens are unavoidable, dim them and use blue-light filters—but think of those as backups, not solutions.

Pairing screen limits with a consistent bedtime and no late-night snacking further supports overnight recovery. Turning off screens isn't about discipline for its own sake. It's about creating the conditions your body and your liver need to reset, repair, and function at their best.

165

TRY NOT TO EAT MIDNIGHT SNACKS

Midnight snacks may feel harmless, but they quietly work against your liver health. The liver, like your gut, is designed to shift from digestion to repair overnight. Eating late at night forces it back into calorie processing mode, interrupting fat breakdown, detox pathways, and insulin regulation. Your gut hormones, ghrelin and leptin, have a circadian rhythm, and late-night snacking disrupts this, which can lead to overeating and feeling less energetic the next day.

Late-night eating is especially rough when snacks are sugary or refined. Blood sugar rises when the body expects rest, pushing insulin higher and encouraging fat storage in the liver. Over time, this pattern increases inflammation and makes it harder for the liver to clear accumulated fat, even if daytime eating looks reasonable.

Timing matters as much as food quality. Giving the liver a clear fasting window, ideally 3 hours between your last meal and sleep, allows metabolic cleanup to happen as intended. People often notice better sleep, improved morning energy, and reduced cravings when late snacking stops.

If nighttime hunger keeps showing up, review your day's journey. Skipping protein earlier in the day, eating too little at dinner, and chronic stress can all drive late cravings. Adjusting those factors is far more effective than willpower at midnight.

Letting the kitchen close at night isn't about restriction; it's about aligning eating with your body's natural rhythms so the liver can focus on repair instead of round-the-clock digestion.

166

CREATE A SLEEP SANCTUARY

Create a sleep sanctuary by making your bedroom feel like a place to shut down, not stay switched on. Your liver does its best repair work while you sleep, but it can't do much if your room feels noisy, bright, or mentally busy.

To create your sanctuary, start with the basics:

- Make your room dark. Streetlights, hallway glow, and alarm clocks all interfere with deep sleep more than people realize. Use blackout curtains or a simple sleep mask if needed. Keep the room a little cooler too, as cooler air helps your body relax and stay asleep, whereas a warmer temperature may impair your ability to fall asleep.
- Clear the distractions and move your phone off the bed or out of arm's reach. Late-night scrolling keeps your brain alert when it should be winding down.
- If there's a TV in the room, turn it off earlier and keep it off overnight.
- Make comfort nonnegotiable and ensure you use pillows that support your neck, sheets that breathe, and bedding that feels good when you climb in. If your pillow is not working for you, know that you can try out pillows and mattresses at stores that sell these items. These small details matter more than expensive gadgets.

Protect what your bedroom is for—rest and relaxation. Don't work, argue, or stress in bed. Train your brain to associate that space with rest. When sleep improves, recovery improves, and your liver finally gets the quiet time it needs to reset.

167

LOWER CORTISOL

Lower your cortisol if you want your liver to work better. Know that constant stress keeps cortisol elevated, and when that hormone stays high, your liver and your metabolism take the hit. High cortisol pushes blood sugar up, increases insulin resistance, and tells your body to store fat, much of it ending up in the liver.

Start lowering your cortisol by slowing things down on purpose. You don't need a "perfect" routine or a silent retreat. Take a few minutes each day to step away from noise and urgency. Go for a short walk, breathe deeply, or sit quietly without your phone, and consider meditation before you get into bed or while you are between your sheets. These small pauses signal to your nervous system that it's time to stand down.

Pay attention to how you start and end your day. Rushing in the morning or scrolling late at night keeps stress hormones elevated around the clock. Create simple bookends instead: Wake up without immediately checking your phone, and wind down before bed with something calming.

Support your body physically and eat regular meals with enough protein and fiber, move your body gently most days, and get consistent sleep. Skipped meals, overtraining, and poor sleep all drive cortisol higher.

You don't have to eliminate stress to protect your liver, you just have to stop living in constant fight-or-flight. Lower cortisol, improve metabolic balance, and give your liver a fighting chance to do its job well.

168

BANISH BLUE LIGHT BEFORE SLEEP

Banish blue light exposure before sleep if you want to help prime your liver to start its repair work. Blue light is the high-energy light emitted from phones, tablets, TVs, and LED bulbs. During the day it helps keep you alert, but at night it sends the wrong signal to your body. Blue light tells your brain it's still daytime, delaying melatonin and cutting into the deep sleep your liver relies on to repair and reset.

Here are some ideas to try:

- **Set a clear screen time cutoff.** Power down your devices at least an hour before bed. This isn't about perfection—it's about giving your body a chance to shift into rest mode. The earlier the screens go off, the easier it is to fall asleep and stay asleep.
- **Change your lighting in the evening.** Use lamps instead of overhead lights and choose warmer, softer bulbs. Bright white light late at night keeps your nervous system switched on and your stress hormones elevated.
- **If screens are unavoidable, reduce the damage.** Lower brightness, activate night mode, and keep devices out of your face. Think of these as backup plans, not solutions.

Pair these habits with a calm bedtime routine and no late-night eating. Remove blue light, protect melatonin, and improve sleep depth. When sleep improves, your liver gets the uninterrupted time it needs to manage fat, regulate blood sugar, and recover properly overnight.

169

BALANCE MELATONIN NATURALLY

Balance your melatonin naturally to support both sleep quality and improve liver function. Melatonin is not only a regulator of sleep–wake cycles, but it also plays a role in metabolic timing, antioxidant activity, and nighttime liver repair. When melatonin release is delayed or suppressed, the liver remains in a daytime metabolic state longer than intended, reducing efficiency of fat oxidation and detoxification processes.

Whenever possible, anchor your melatonin production with proper light exposure and obtain natural daylight early in the morning to synchronize circadian rhythms and promote appropriate melatonin secretion later in the evening. In contrast, excessive exposure to artificial light at night—especially blue-spectrum light—suppresses melatonin and disrupts circadian signaling to the liver. In addition, late-night eating interferes with melatonin release and prolongs hepatic glucose production and insulin activity. Finishing meals at least 2 to 3 hours before sleep allows the liver to transition from nutrient processing to repair and metabolic maintenance.

Maintaining consistent sleep and wake times gives your body a stable, predictable routine. Irregular schedules impair melatonin amplitude and timing, leading to fragmented sleep and metabolic dysregulation.

Melatonin supplementation is not required for most individuals. Instead, you should regulate your melatonin naturally by supporting endogenous production through light management, meal timing, and sleep regularity. These actions will strengthen circadian alignment and allow the liver to carry out essential overnight recovery functions more effectively.

HYDRATE SMARTLY BEFORE BED

Hydrate smartly before bed to support overnight recovery without disrupting sleep and needing to get up to visit the bathroom. Adequate hydration is necessary for liver function, including blood filtration, nutrient transport, and toxin clearance. However, excessive fluid intake late at night can fragment sleep, which ultimately undermines the liver's ability to perform repair and metabolic regulation during overnight hours.

Front-load your hydration earlier in the day. Consuming most fluids in the morning and afternoon supports plasma volume and cellular hydration without increasing nighttime awakenings. As evening approaches, reduce large amounts of fluid and shift toward smaller, measured sips if needed.

In addition, pay attention to *what* you drink. Alcohol dehydrates and directly impairs liver metabolism, while sugary beverages increase hepatic glucose load and insulin demand. Caffeine late in the day delays sleep onset and alters circadian signaling. If it is late in the day, it is best to consume plain water or mineral water as the most supportive option.

Consider electrolyte balance rather than volume alone. Inadequate sodium or mineral intake can trigger thirst late at night, leading to overconsumption of fluids before bed. Another not so uncommon event is leg cramps, which can also occur due to electrolyte abnormalities. Balanced meals earlier in the day help stabilize fluid regulation.

You should aim to stop significant fluid intake 60–90 minutes before sleep, as this protects sleep continuity, supports circadian-driven liver processes, and allows the body to focus on repair rather than nighttime disruption.

171

DON'T OVERDO CAFFEINE

Don't overdo caffeine if you want to protect both your energy levels and liver health. In excess, caffeine increases metabolic demand, elevates cortisol, and interferes with sleep—reducing the liver's ability to carry out overnight repair and fat metabolism.

That being said, moderate caffeine intake has documented liver benefits. Regular coffee consumption has been associated with lower liver enzyme levels and reduced risk of fatty liver disease, fibrosis, and cirrhosis, and is associated with reduced risk of liver cancer. These effects are thought to come from caffeine itself, along with coffee's polyphenols, which support antioxidant activity and improve insulin sensitivity. In reasonable amounts, caffeine can enhance fat oxidation and reduce hepatic inflammation.

The line toward liver damage is crossed when your caffeine dose or timing is off. Large amounts and late-day caffeine disrupt sleep architecture, shortening deep sleep and impairing circadian signaling to the liver. Even if total sleep time seems adequate, recovery quality suffers. Use caffeine deliberately; keep intake earlier in the day, ideally with food; and avoid stacking multiple sources. Pay attention to how your body responds rather than chasing stimulation.

Caffeine can support liver health when used wisely; however, it is important to respect the dose, protect sleep, and allow the liver to benefit from caffeine's protective effects without paying the price of overuse.

172

COOL TEMPERATURES HELP SLEEP

Cooler temperatures help sleep by supporting the body's natural thermoregulation and circadian biology. Core body temperature is meant to drop in the evening, and this decline is a key signal that initiates sleep onset. When the sleeping environment is too warm, this process is delayed, resulting in lighter, more fragmented sleep that reduces overnight recovery.

Lower ambient temperatures promote deeper slow-wave sleep, the stage most closely associated with physical repair and metabolic regulation. During this phase, the liver increases fat oxidation, regulates glucose output, and supports detoxification pathways. Heat stress interferes with these processes by elevating cortisol and increasing nighttime awakenings, which leads to poor overall sleep and rest.

Aim to keep your bedroom cool, generally between 60°F and 67°F (16°C and 19°C), a range supported by sleep research for optimal sleep quality. Individual comfort varies, but slightly cooler than daytime temperatures is consistently beneficial. Breathable bedding and moisture-wicking fabrics further support heat dissipation during the night. Cooling pads are also now available and even zoned for half a bed if your sleeping partner prefers a different temperature from you.

Avoid behaviors that raise body temperature close to bedtime, such as heavy meals, alcohol, and intense exercise late in the evening. These things delay the natural cooling response and disrupt your sleep architecture. A warm shower earlier in the evening can help by triggering a rebound cooling effect afterward.

Support your body's temperature drop, deepen sleep, and create the conditions your liver needs to perform essential overnight repair and metabolic functions.

173

ALIGN SLEEP WITH CIRCADIAN RHYTHM

Align your sleep with circadian rhythms to support your metabolic health and liver function. Circadian rhythms are internal 24-hour biological clocks that regulate sleep, hormone release, glucose metabolism, and liver enzyme activity. When your sleep timing is misaligned, meaning you are sleeping at irregular hours or against the light–dark cycle, these systems fall out of sync, increasing insulin resistance, inflammation, and fat accumulation in the liver.

The liver is particularly sensitive to circadian disruption. Many hepatic genes involved in detoxification and lipid metabolism follow time-dependent patterns. Consistent sleep and wake times help preserve this timing and improve overnight metabolic efficiency.

Anchor your schedule whenever possible. Wake at the same time daily, even on nonworkdays, to stabilize circadian signaling. Use morning light exposure to reinforce daytime alertness, and limit evening light to allow melatonin to rise. Keep meals aligned with waking hours, and avoid eating during the biological night.

For shift workers, prioritize consistency over clock time. Maintain the same sleep schedule across workdays and days off when feasible. Use bright light during work shifts to support alertness, then minimize light exposure after work with sunglasses and blackout curtains. Create a cool, dark, quiet sleep environment during daytime rest.

When traveling across time zones, adjust light exposure deliberately. Seek daylight in the new morning, avoid light late at night, and shift meals toward local time as soon as possible. Strategic light management helps reset circadian rhythms and reduces metabolic strain on the liver.

174

RESET YOUR LIVER BY SAYING NO

Reset your liver by saying no: no to constant stimulation, no to late nights, and no to habits that keep your body stuck in overdrive. The liver depends on predictable rhythms to regulate glucose, process fats, and carry out overnight detoxification. When stress, late eating and poor sleep become the norm, those rhythms break down.

Saying no to these bad habits reduces physiological load. Chronic overcommitment elevates cortisol, increases insulin resistance, and pushes more fat toward the liver. Late nights and irregular schedules disrupt circadian signaling, leaving the liver in a perpetual daytime metabolic state when it should be repairing.

To protect your liver health:

- **Say no to late meals.** Eating close to bedtime keeps insulin high and delays the liver's transition into fat-burning and cleanup mode.
- **Say no to endless screen time at night.** Late-night screen time suppresses melatonin and fragments sleep.
- **Say no to using caffeine or sugar to power through.** This forces the liver to compensate for depleted energy systems.
- **Say no to alcohol when recovery matters.** Alcohol is a direct liver toxin that halts fat metabolism and detox pathways until it is fully processed, even at moderate levels.

Saying no isn't about restriction, it's about recovery. Each boundary you set lowers inflammatory pressure and restores metabolic timing. Create space for sleep, regular meals, and mental downtime. When you reduce constant demand, the liver regains its natural rhythm and can focus on repair instead of survival.

175

RESET YOUR LIVER BY SAYING YES

Reset your liver by saying yes to signals that reinforce metabolic and circadian stability. The liver is a central metabolic organ whose functions are broad and include glucose regulation, lipid processing, bile production, and detoxification, all of which are tightly regulated by circadian clocks and hormonal cues. When these signals are consistent, hepatic efficiency improves and inflammatory burden decreases.

To protect your liver health:

- **Say yes to consistent sleep timing.** Stable sleep–wake cycles strengthen central and peripheral circadian clocks, including the liver clock that regulates time-dependent gene expression involved in fat oxidation and insulin sensitivity. Deep, consolidated sleep supports nocturnal liver repair.
- **Say yes to aligned meal timing.** Eating earlier in the evening reduces nocturnal insulin exposure. Time-restricted eating windows have been shown to improve liver fat content and metabolic flexibility by allowing predictable fasting periods.
- **Say yes to light management.** Morning light exposure suppresses daytime melatonin and reinforces circadian alignment, while reduced evening light allows melatonin to rise. Melatonin supports antioxidant defense and helps signal the liver to transition into nighttime metabolic mode.
- **Say yes to regular, moderate movement.** Low- to moderate-intensity activity improves insulin signaling and reduces hepatic fat accumulation without elevating stress hormones.

When inputs align with circadian and metabolic physiology, the liver shifts from compensatory stress to efficient repair and long-term resilience.

176

FACTOR MENOPAUSE INTO LIVER HEALTH

If you are female, you need to factor menopause into your liver health, because hormonal shifts change how the liver manages fat, glucose, and inflammation. As estrogen levels decline during perimenopause and menopause, the liver becomes more prone to fat accumulation and insulin resistance. Estrogen normally helps regulate lipid metabolism and supports healthy bile flow, so its loss alters hepatic function even when diet and weight stay the same.

Lower estrogen shifts fat storage toward the abdomen and liver. This increases the risk of nonalcoholic fatty liver disease and worsens blood sugar control. At the same time, changes in cortisol sensitivity during menopause can amplify stress responses, further increasing liver fat and inflammatory signaling.

Sleep disruption is another major factor. Hot flashes, night sweats, and fragmented sleep interfere with circadian rhythms that govern liver enzyme activity and overnight repair. Poor sleep raises insulin resistance and limits fat oxidation, placing additional strain on the liver.

Support the transition deliberately. Prioritize protein and fiber to stabilize blood sugar, maintain regular meal timing to protect circadian alignment, and engage in resistance and low-impact aerobic exercise to preserve insulin sensitivity. Manage stress and protect sleep aggressively, as both have outsized metabolic effects during menopause.

Menopause changes the metabolic landscape. Aligning sleep, nutrition, stress management, and movement with this new hormonal environment is key to supporting long-term liver health.

177

EMBRACE FASTING

Embrace fasting to support liver metabolism and cellular repair. Periods without food allow the liver to shift from constant nutrient processing into maintenance mode. During fasting, hepatic insulin levels fall, glycogen stores are depleted, and the liver increases fat oxidation and autophagy—processes essential for reducing liver fat and clearing damaged cellular components.

Fasting improves metabolic flexibility. By extending the time between meals, the liver becomes better at switching between glucose and fat as fuel. This shift lowers triglyceride accumulation in the liver and improves insulin sensitivity, even without changes in total calorie intake.

Start with time, not deprivation. A daily fasting window of 12–14 hours is often enough to produce benefits, especially when the fast occurs overnight. Finishing dinner earlier and avoiding late-night snacks allows the liver to follow its natural circadian rhythm and prioritize repair during sleep.

The quality of your food still matters, and fasting does not cancel out poor food choices. Balanced meals with adequate protein, fiber, and healthy fats support stable blood sugar and make fasting easier and more sustainable. It is also important to avoid sabotaging your fast with intake of ultra-processed foods and high-fructose corn syrup–containing items.

Fasting is a tool, not a stress test. Excessive restriction can raise cortisol and backfire metabolically. Use fasting to create predictable recovery periods, reduce liver workload, and reinforce the timing signals that support long-term liver health.

178

GET YOUR MORNING SUN

Get morning sun to set your internal clock and support liver health. Early daylight exposure is one of the strongest signals for aligning circadian rhythms, which regulate hormone release, metabolism, and liver enzyme activity. When light hits the eyes in the morning, it suppresses melatonin and triggers a cortisol rise that helps the body transition into an active metabolic state.

This timing matters for the liver. Proper circadian alignment improves insulin sensitivity and regulates hepatic glucose production throughout the day. When morning light is missed, especially with late nights or indoor lifestyles, circadian rhythms drift, increasing the risk of blood sugar dysregulation and liver fat accumulation.

Aim for natural light within 30–60 minutes of waking. Even 5–15 minutes outdoors can be effective, and longer exposure on cloudy days helps compensate for lower light intensity. Avoid sunglasses during this time if it's safe to do so, as light needs to reach the eyes to signal the brain.

Morning light also improves sleep later that night. By anchoring the start of the circadian day, melatonin rises earlier and more predictably in the evening, supporting deeper sleep and overnight liver repair.

Make morning sun a daily habit. It's simple, free, and one of the most powerful ways to support metabolic rhythm and liver function.

179

SCHEDULE GRATITUDE AND REST DAYS

Use gratitude and rest days as intentional tools to support liver repair, because both influence physiology more than most people realize. Liver health depends on signals of safety and recovery. Gratitude lowers psychological stress, and rest days reduce physiological strain. When stress is lowered and recovery is prioritized, the liver shifts from constant defense into repair, reinforcing the idea that healing is built through consistency, not extremes.

Chronic psychological stress activates the hypothalamic–pituitary–adrenal (HPA) axis, leading to sustained cortisol release. Elevated cortisol increases hepatic glucose production, worsens insulin resistance, and promotes fat accumulation in the liver. Over time, this stress-driven metabolic state increases inflammation and oxidative burden on liver cells.

Gratitude practices help interrupt this cycle. Research shows that gratitude activates the parasympathetic nervous system and reduces activity in stress-related brain regions, leading to lower cortisol levels and improved heart rate. These shifts support better sleep quality and reduce inflammation, creating conditions that favor hepatic fat oxidation, antioxidant activity, and nighttime cellular repair.

Rest days play a similar role on the physical side. Continuous high-intensity exercise without adequate recovery elevates cortisol and increases muscle-derived inflammatory signals that the liver must help clear. Strategic rest allows these markers to normalize, improves insulin sensitivity, and reduces hepatic workload. During recovery periods, the liver can redirect energy toward glycogen replenishment, detoxification pathways, and tissue repair.

INDEX

ABOUT THE AUTHOR

SUPRIYA JOSHI, MD, is a gastroenterologist and hepatologist at Trillium Health Partners; an assistant professor at the University of Toronto's Temerty Faculty of Medicine; and the current medical director at West GTA Endoscopy. She is also medical director, advisor, and board member of Fatty Liver Alliance, an organization promoting public advocacy and education with global reach. Passionate about lifestyle-based liver care, Dr. Joshi completed executive education in sustainable nutrition at Harvard University and Coaching Essentials for Healthcare Professionals through Temerty Faculty of Medicine, University of Toronto.

With more than twenty years of clinical experience, she is frequently invited to speak on liver disease, has appeared as a guest on many podcasts, and is the founder of the social media public education platform @LiverHealthMD. When she educates, her aim is to empower people to pivot and learn the tools that can optimize their health journey while preventing chronic metabolic disease. Learn about Dr. Joshi's master class and coaching services at LiverHealthMD.com. Outside of caring for her patients, she walks the talk, is a fitness enthusiast, and cherishes spending time with her family.